WITHDRAWN

Samantha Taylor

BEAUTY THERAPY

edition

D0452919

earsonschoolsandfe.co.uk

✓ Free online support
✓ Useful weblinks
✓ 24 hour online ordering

0845 630 44 44

Heinemann
Part of Pearson

Heinemann is an imprint of Pearson Education Limited, a company incorporated in England and Wales, having its registered office at Edinburgh Gate, Harlow, Essex, CM20 2JE. Registered company number: 872828

www.pearsonschoolsandfecolleges.co.uk

Heinemann is a registered trademark of Pearson Education Limited

Text © Samantha Taylor, 2004, 2010

This second edition first published 2010

12 11 10

10 9 8 7 6 5 4 3 2 1

British Library Cataloguing in Publication Data

A catalogue record for this book is available from the British Library

ISBN 978 0 435 02658 5

Edited by Caroline Broughton
Designed by Dickidot Limited
Typeset by Dickidot Limited
Original illustrations © Pearson Education 2010
Illustrated by Artful Doodlers
Cover design by Wooden Ark
Picture research by Suzi Paz
Cover photo/illustration © Imagesource
Printed in the UK by Scotprint

Websites

There are links to relevant websites in this book. In order to ensure that the links are up to date, that the links work, and that the sites are not inadvertently linked to sites that could be considered offensive, we have made the links available on our website at www.pearsonhotlinks.co.uk. Search for the title Level 1 (NVQ/SVQ) Certificate in Beauty Therapy Candidate Handbook or ISBN 9780435026585.

Contents

Acknowledgements

The author and publisher would like to thank the following individuals and organisations for permission to reproduce photographs:

Yuri Arcurs/Shutterstock p 2, p 203; Science Photo Library / Cordelia Molloy p 6; Carlton Professional p 21/131; Rade Kovac/Shutterstock p 27; Imagesource p 28; Payless Images/Shutterstock p 50; Jason Stitt/Shutterstock p 66, p 205 (young skin); Kim Karpeles / Alamy p 68; Shopics / Alamy p 70; Solovieva Ekaterina/Shutterstock p 92; DR P. MARAZZI / SCIENCE PHOTO LIBRARY p 108 (impetigo, conjunctivitis, bruising), p 109 (scar tissue, eczema), p 170 (scabies), p 171 (swelling and inflammation, discoloured nails, damaged nails); ST BARTHOLOMEW'S HOSPITAL / SCIENCE PHOTO LIBRARY p 108 (cold sores); IAN HOOTON / SCIENCE PHOTO LIBRARY p 109 (recent sunburn); JANE SHEMILT / SCIENCE PHOTO LIBRARY p 109/170 (cuts and grazes); Alena Ozerova/Shutterstock p 128; Apollofoto/Shutterstock p 139 (normal skin); Monkey Business Images/Shutterstock p v, p 139 (dry skin); Shutterstock/Valua Vitaly p 144; Marc Dietrich/Shutterstock p 156; Science Photo Library p 170 (warts, ringworm); DR M.A. ANSARY / SCIENCE PHOTO LIBRARY p171 (overgrown cuticles); Vibrant Image Studio/Shutterstock p 198; Darren Hubley/Shutterstock p 209; Junial Enterprises/Shutterstock p 214; Gregor Schuster/PhotographersChoice/GettyImages p 95.

All other photos: Pearson Education Ltd/Stuart Cox; Pearson Education Ltd/Gareth Boden; Pearson Education Ltd/Mindstudio; Pearson Education Ltd/Jules Selmes; Pearson Education Ltd/Studio 8/Clark Wiseman.

Every effort has been made to contact copyright holders of material reproduced in this book. Any omissions will be rectified in subsequent printings if notice is given to the publishers.

Crown copyright material reproduced with permission of the Controller of Her Majesty's Stationery Office and the Queen's Printer for Scotland.

iv

Introduction

Why choose a career in beauty therapy?

Beauty therapy offers opportunity and choice throughout your working life. Once you have qualified and gained your skills you can take them wherever you want, whenever you want. If you are thinking about a career in beauty therapy, you could be using your skills while cruising the world on a luxury liner, working as a make-up artist, or running your own beauty salon business. The opportunities in the beauty industry are amazing, but you must be prepared to work hard and show dedication to the industry. If you are ready to do this, you will have the opportunity for new and exciting experiences.

 Salon life

Jasmina completed her NVQ Level 1 Beauty Therapy before moving on to complete Levels 2 and 3. She is now working on a cruise liner carrying out beauty and complementary therapies on the passengers. Her days are very long but very rewarding as she gets to see lots of exciting countries and the chance to mix with many different people. Jasmina has decided that her next career move should be trying for a job as an airline therapist as she has got the travel bug and fancies travelling around the world while working in a job she loves.

Jasmina

What is a Certificate/Diploma (NVQ/SVQ)?

Certificate/Diploma (NVQs/SVQs) are qualifications based on the skills and knowledge that you will need at work, so if you want to get a recognised qualification related to an industry or sector an NVQ/SVQ could be for you. You can study in a variety of places and in different ways such as at work, in college or school, or as part of an apprenticeship.

NVQ stands for National Vocational Qualification and SVQ for Scottish Vocational Qualification. They are 'competence-based' qualifications, which means that you learn practical skills designed to help you develop the skills and knowledge to do a job well.

NVQs/SVQs in Beauty Therapy can be studied at Levels 1 (Certificate), 2 and 3 (Diploma).

Progression

Usually if starting at the beginning, you will come in at Level 1 or 2, but this depends on your GCSE results and the requirements requested by the course provider.

After completing your Level 1 (NVQ/SVQ) Certificate in Beauty Therapy it is best to study further in order to gain Level 2 (NVQ/SVQ) Diploma; this could be in Beauty Therapy or Hairdressing, the choice is yours.

How do I gain a Level 1 Certificate (NVQ/SVQ)?

The Level 1 Certificate (NVQ/SVQ) in Beauty therapy involves **three** mandatory units that **must** be completed to achieve the qualification, and four optional units from which you need to choose **two** to go with your mandatory units.

Mandatory Units

G20 Make sure your own actions reduce risks to health and safety

G3 Contribute to the development of effective working relationships

B1 Prepare and maintain salon treatment work areas

Optional Units

G2 Assist with salon reception duties

B2 Assist with facial skin care treatments

B3 Assist with day make-up

N1 Assist with nail services

NVQ/SVQ structure

All NVQ/SVQs have the same structure, which includes:

- **Units.** These are the subjects that you will be learning about. For example, when learning about reception skills for Level 1, the unit is called: Unit G2 Assist with salon reception duties.

- **Elements.** Each unit is made up of elements. For example, Unit G2 Assist with salon reception duties is made up of: Maintain the reception area; Attend to clients and enquiries; Help to make appointments for salon services.

- **Performance criteria.** These describe the activities, either theory or practical, that need to be carried out by you in order to complete the unit successfully.

- **Range statements.** These are the situations that must be covered in your learning, for example, the type of client, type of treatment or booking method (e.g. phone or face-to-face).

- **Knowledge and understanding.** This is the background knowledge that you must know so that you can carry out the treatment or activity competently.

- **Evidence.** Evidence is proof of your learning. It can be coursework, assignments, client letters, drawings, photos or tutor comments. Most evidence will be signed by your assessor, to confirm that it is correct and your own work.

All of these need to be gathered in a portfolio to show proof of your learning and progress.

Assessment – How you will be assessed

Practical: For each unit that you practise your skills in you will need to be assessed. Usually this will be through observation of your practical skills by your assessor, and if you prove that you are safe and competent you will pass the assessments.

Theory: You will also need to keep a portfolio of evidence; this will be a file containing information to show that you have covered all of the necessary knowledge requirements to be able to carry out your practical skills. This will be recorded in a candidate log book which will be signed by an assessor.

As well as your practical assessments and portfolio of evidence you will need to do assignments and sit tests on various units for your qualification.

How to use this book

Level 1 (NVQ/SVQ) Certificate in Beauty Therapy Candidate Handbook will introduce you to the basics of beauty therapy and covers all the necessary performance and criteria statements for NVQ1 Beauty Therapy. It has been organised into three sections: 1: In the workplace, 2: Practical skills and 3: Anatomy and physiology, and has been written to cover all the units within the new standards for 2010. Each unit has been structured to follow the main learning outcomes for that unit.

You will come across the following features which will support your learning:

Key terms: Definition of key terms at the start of each unit.

Top tip boxes: Helpful information about good practice or useful suggestions.

Get up and go: Activities to do as projects, homework, discussions or group work.

Salon stories: Examples of real-life situations that could happen in a salon.

Memory joggers: Questions at the end of each element or topic to help you recall information and show what you have learned.

Get ahead: Extension activities to push you forward in your studies.

Saks

We are pleased that this book has been endorsed by SAKS. Saks Education is officially acknowledged as the UK's Best Training Provider, having been awarded Beacon Status by the Quality Improvement Agency and all grade ones by the Adult Learning Inspectorate for providing outstanding training. It is the only hair and beauty work-based learning provider to have been awarded both accolades.

Saks recognise that education is the key to success! A good sound education can lead to numerous career opportunities within the beauty industry and your Level 1 (NVQ/SVQ) Certificate is the first step on the path to becoming a successful beauty therapist.

Top tips

Points to think about when putting your portfolio together:

1 Does it have an attractive front cover, e.g. magazine cuttings, clear bold writing, and lots of colour and design?

2 Does it have an organised, easy-to-understand contents page and clear page numbers throughout?

3 Does it contain clear and neat notes from each lesson, either handwritten or word-processed?

4 Does it include interesting articles on health and beauty subjects?

5 Does it contain a conclusion – your comments at the end of the portfolio on:
- what you learned or gained from the course
- how much you enjoyed the course
- whether you are intending to progress further to Level 2
- any other information you think might be useful?

UNIT G20

Make sure your own actions reduce risks to health and safety

Beauty therapy is an exciting, fast-moving industry, but just as it presents you with some great opportunities, it also involves responsibilities. As a beauty therapist, you will be working with clients and using certain tools and products, and there are procedures that you must follow in order to ensure that your actions do not create any health and safety hazards and that you do not ignore hazards that present risks in your workplace.

Your health and safety responsibilities at work include making sure that your actions protect the health and safety of you and others, meet any legal responsibilities and follow workplace instructions.

In this unit you will learn about:

- Identifying the hazards and evaluating the risks in your workplace
- Health and safety laws
- Workplace policies
- Personal presentation and behaviour

2

Here are some key terms you will meet in this unit:

Hazard – something with the potential to cause harm

Risk – the likelihood that a hazard will actually cause harm

Control – how risks are identified, managed and then reduced to acceptable levels

Legislation – a law or laws passed by an official body

Negligence – carelessness and lack of attention

Fire risk assessment – a formal check to identify what the dangers of fire are and what can be done to prevent a fire

Assembly point – an agreed meeting place outside a building

Premises – a place of business

Health and Safety Executive (HSE) – the government body that is in charge of making the rules governing health and safety

Disinfection – use of a chemical that cuts down bacteria and micro-organisms

Sterilisation – a procedure that kills micro-organisms

Evacuate – leave an area or premises in an orderly fashion

Flammable – something that can very easily catch fire

Precautions – things you can do in advance to stop something happening

Cross-infection – when germs or bacteria are transferred from one person to another

Identifying the hazards and evaluating the risks in your workplace

This unit covers the health and safety responsibilities for everyone in the beauty therapy industry. As a beauty therapist you have to be aware of specific **legislation** for your particular job role. The Health and Safety at Work Act (HASWA) 1974 (see page 6 for more information) covers everyone in the salon, and it is important that you know and understand your responsibilities under this act. You must always make sure that your actions do not create a health and safety risk. In the workplace, many things can cause accidents, injury or illness if they are not recognised and made safe.

Risk assessment and control

Risk assessment and control are the responsibility of everyone and any health and safety risks you spot should be reported immediately. For your own safety, you cannot always act upon the risk, and in such cases you will have to inform a higher authority so that it can be dealt with.

It is crucial that you understand the terms 'hazard', 'risk' and 'control'.

- A **hazard** is something with the potential to cause harm; something that could cause an accident or injury.
- A **risk** is the likelihood that the hazard will actually cause harm; the threat of something dangerous happening because of the hazard.
- **Control** refers to the measures that you put into place to remove risks or to reduce them to acceptable levels.

Almost anything may be a hazard, but may or may not become a risk. Some hazards could be thought of as 'accidents waiting to happen', as they pose such a high risk. Other hazards are less of a risk, but need to be identified and controlled nevertheless.

For example, in a beauty salon, many deliveries are made. If some boxes of skin care products were delivered and set down on the floor beside reception, these boxes would be a **hazard**. The **risk** would be the chance that someone could trip over the boxes and hurt themselves. The risk would be high if the boxes were in the middle of the floor, directly in the path of the therapists and clients in the salon, but the risk could be **controlled** by moving the boxes to a place where they are less likely to be in the way of people who are moving about in the salon.

You need to be aware of the hazards that may exist in your workplace, and you will need to be able to spot hazards, identify the risks that they pose, and take steps to make sure that they do not cause a problem to you, your clients or other staff.

>> **Get up and go!**

On page 5 is a table giving you examples of hazards which present risks. Read the table of hazards and risks and, for each situation, complete the table by stating how you would make it safer and less likely to turn into an accident or injury, i.e. how you would control the risk.

4

Hazard	Risk	Control measure
Electrical leads trailing on the floor	Tripping over leads	Run flexes alongside the wall
A light bulb that has blown	Accidents because of poor light	
Highly polished floors	Slipping	
Badly fitting carpet or lino	Tripping up	
Trolleys and desks overloaded with equipment and products	Furniture tipping over	
Plugs that have loose or frayed leads	Possible electric shock or risk of fire	
Rushing about too much, without concentrating	Bumping into people and causing an injury	
A therapist carrying tools in the pocket of her uniform	Cuts or wounds if someone bumps into her	
Carrying too much at once	Can't see where you are going which results in an accident or a bad back	
Breakages or spills that are not cleared up instantly	Cuts or slipping over	
Unsterilised tools	**Cross-infection**	

Remember that you will not be able to deal with all hazards yourself. Work within the limits of your own authority and if you are unable to deal with a problem, report it and be clear and concise in your information to the person who is responsible. Do not ignore it, hoping it will go away, as you may endanger another person.

? Memory jogger

1 Who is responsible for health and safety in the workplace?

2 What do the letters HASWA stand for?

3 What is a risk and what is a hazard? Give two examples of each.

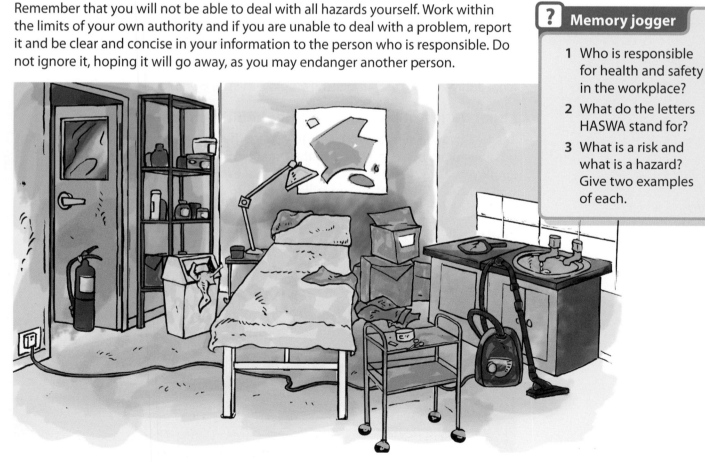

How good are you at spotting a hazard? Identify the hazards in the salon shown and make a list of them. How many did you spot?

Health and safety laws [1]

Every workplace, whether it is a shop, office, factory or beauty salon, must follow a set of health and safety rules laid down by the **Health and Safety Executive (HSE)**. These rules are designed to protect employers, employees and clients from accident, illness and injury. The acts relevant to you are listed below.

- The Health and Safety at Work Act 1974 (HASWA).
- The Fire Precaution Work Place Regulations 1997.
- The Electricity at Work Regulations 1989.
- The Gas Safety (Installation and Use) Regulations 1994.
- The Manual Handling Operations Regulations 1992.
- The Personal Protective Equipment at Work Regulations 1992.
- The Control of Substances Hazardous to Health Regulations 2002 (COSHH).
- The Health and Safety Regulations (First Aid) 1981.
- The Environmental Protection Act 1990, Waste Regulations 1992 and Special Waste Regulations 1996.
- The Reporting of Injuries, Diseases and Dangerous Occurrences Regulations 1995 (RIDDOR).
- The Local Government (Miscellaneous Provisions) Act 1982.

The Health and Safety at Work Act 1974 (HASWA)

This is one of the most important acts that you need to know about. It covers the legal duties of both employers and employees in all workplaces.

Legal duties of employers under health and safety law

The Health and Safety at Work Act 1974 states that an employer must do everything possible to provide a safe and healthy workplace with adequate welfare facilities. Employers have a legal duty to make sure that everyone is kept healthy, safe and well at work. It is a legal duty to follow these and if a business is found negligent it can be prosecuted.

Carrying out regular checks on electrical equipment to make sure that it is in safe working order is one of the responsibilities of employer to employee

Legal duties of employees under health and safety law

The **HSE** (Health and Safety Executive, the government body that makes the rules regarding health and safety) also expects all employees to play their part in taking reasonable care of their own and others' health and safety. Your responsibilities are outlined in the Health and Safety Law poster. Failure to follow the act can result in serious consequences and you should be aware that heavy fines and/or imprisonment can result if the act is ignored. If you have any worries about healthy and safety, talk them through with someone more senior. Make sure that your concerns are recorded, and any action required is followed up.

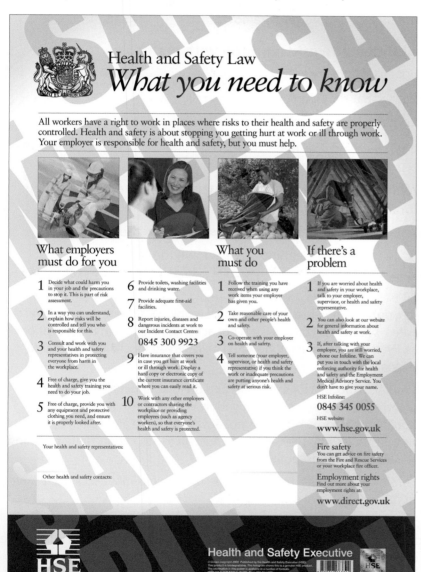

The Health and Safety Law poster (Source: Health and Safety Executive)

 Top tip

For further information visit the Health and Safety Executive website. You can access this by going to www.pearsonhotlinks.co.uk and searching for this title.

 Get ahead

Search the Internet to find out about any beauty therapy businesses that have been fined or prosecuted because they have not followed the Health and Safety at Work Act. The businesses could include salons, spas, product retailers, product manufacturers and so on.

7

Health and safety laws (2)

Hot and cold running water

The salon must have a constant supply of hot and cold running water. Each treatment room should have a separate sink with hot and cold running water. However, if a large treatment room has been separated into treatment bays by curtains, then a central sink will do.

The water supply is used for sanitising hands and tools, cleaning the room, and for parts of the treatment, for example, mask removal.

Top tip ✓

Dirty water smells unpleasant and encourages the growth of bacteria, which can cause illness.

Your responsibilities at work: working with water

Report to your supervisor *immediately*:

- blocked sinks, so that they don't overflow
- water that comes out of the tap a funny colour
- any leak, loose tap or cracked pipe.

Don't:

- leave taps running, especially the hot water tap as this is wasteful and very expensive for the salon
- flush mask products or other semi-solid products down the sink
- pour chemicals, solvents or cleaning agents down the sink.

Staff areas

Your employer has a duty to provide a space in which employees can rest and eat. A staff room or separate area is important because it is not acceptable to eat in the reception or treatment areas. Even drinks in the salon should be reserved for clients, in order to maintain a professional image.

The staff room should have an area for staff coats and preferably lockers for valuables such as handbags and expensive beauty therapy tools. A separate toilet and washing facility would also be ideal, but this is not always possible and staff may have to share the toilet with clients. If this is the case, staff must give their clients preference and make sure that they leave the room spotless at all times.

A staff area with comfortable seating, tea- and coffee-making facilities and a microwave would also benefit the well-being of staff.

In the beauty industry, you are there to provide a service to clients, so there is not much time to relax and unwind. If you work in a successful salon, you will be rushed off your feet. The area that your employer provides for your rest periods is therefore very important.

The Reporting of Injuries, Diseases and Dangerous Occurences Regulations 1995 (RIDDOR)

Under these regulations, the employer must send a report to the local authority if:

- anyone dies or is seriously injured at work
- anyone is absent from work for more than three days because of a diagnosed disease or accident connected with work.

Reporting accidents

Although not all accidents must be reported to the local authority, all accidents and injuries must nevertheless be reported to the relevant person. If a workplace employs more than ten staff then by law it must have an accident book. This can be bought from a stationery shop and must be kept somewhere that is easy for all staff to access. The Data Protection Act states that an employee's information must be kept secure and private. Therefore, once the completed sheet is removed from the accident book, it should be passed to the relevant person to be filed in a lockable cabinet. If your salon is small with less than ten employees, it is still a good idea for the employer to keep a record of all accidents and injuries.

ACCIDENT REPORT FORM

SECTION 1 PERSONAL DETAILS

Full name of first aider/staff member: _____

Position held in salon: _____

Date: _____

Accident (injury) ☐   Incident (illness) ☐

Time and date of accident/incident: _____

Full name of injured/ill person: _____

Staff member ☐   Client ☐   Other ☐

Address: _____

Tel. no: _____

SECTION 2 ACCIDENT/INCIDENT DETAILS

Describe what happened. In the case of an accident, state clearly what the injured person was doing: _____

Name and address/tel. no. of witness(es), if any: _____

Action taken

Ambulance called ☐   Taken to hospital ☐   Sent to hospital ☐   First aid given ☐

Taken home ☐   Sent home ☐   Returned to work ☐

SECTION 3 PREVENTATIVE ACTION

Preventative action implemented ☐

Describe action taken: _____

Date implemented: _____

Signature of first aider/staff member: _____

Signature salon manager/owner: _____

Date: _____

A page from an accident book

The information that should be included when reporting an accident is:

- the date and time it happened
- the place/area
- the type of accident, for example, a cut, a fall or a bang on the head, and how it happened
- the name of the injured or ill person
- what first aid was given, if any
- what happened after the accident – whether the person went to hospital, was sent home or returned to work
- the name and signature of the first aider or person who sorted the matter out.

Top tip

If you need to report an accident, act cool and calm and think very carefully about what you need to do.

It is not your responsibility to deal with accidents or give first aid. However, you *must* report to your health and safety supervisor anything that you think might be a danger to the general public and staff. So make sure you know who your supervisor is.

Top tip ✓

Always find out the fire and evacuation procedure for any place in which you work or study. By law an employer, school or college must give you this information straight away. If it has not, make sure that you find out as soon as possible.

Health and safety laws (3)

The Fire Precaution Work Place Regulations 1997

The law says that all workplaces must carry out a **fire risk assessment** and a yearly fire drill. All staff must be trained in the fire drill – what to do in the event of a fire and how to **evacuate** the building safely.

The fire drill

The information that staff should be given about the fire drill includes:

- how to sound the alarm and call for help
- who to report to
- the responsibilities of staff to both clients and the people they work with
- how to leave the building safely
- where the emergency exit is
- where the **assembly point** is.

Your responsibilities at work: fire safety

Do:

- leave all doors unlocked wherever possible
- keep **flammable** products such as aerosols away from heat
- report anything that you think may be a fire hazard – it is better to be safe than sorry.

Don't:

- block doorways and exits
- smoke inside
- warm towels on electric or gas heaters.

Building evacuation procedures in the event of fire or bomb alert

The following procedure has been agreed and must be followed. Any staff member who does not comply is committing an infringement of the college disciplinary code. Whenever a fire occurs, the main consideration is to get everybody out of the building safely. Protection of personal or college property is incidental.

Raising the alarm

Anyone discovering a fire must immediately raise the alarm by operating the nearest fire alarm and report to the controller the fire location.

On hearing the alarm the receptionist will immediately contact the emergency services and then evacuate the building.

In the event of a fire being discovered when the reception is unmanned – the premises officer on duty will contact the emergency services and assume control.

On hearing the alarm

All those in senior positions proceed to the control point, normally at a main entrance to the building – where one person must take control of the proceedings.

All other staff: close windows; switch off machinery and lights, and close doors on leaving the room.

Assist less able colleagues, leave the building by the nearest marked route and proceed quickly to the appropriate assembly point. Staff must supervise their class.

Staff evacuating the building must check their locality is clear.

Assembly points

Everyone must remain at assembly points well away from buildings and clear of access roads.

Report to control in person or via two-way radios where allocated.

Everyone must remain at assembly points until further instructions.

DO NOT re-enter the building until you are told it is safe to do so.

An example of a fire evacuation procedure

≫ **Get up and go!**

What other responsibilities for fire prevention can you think of? Add some more to the do and don't lists, then write them in a table like the one below. In the second column, write down the reason for each action. In other words, write down the hazards then explain what the risks are.

Hazard	Risk
Blocked doorways and exits	
Smoking inside	
Warming towels on electric heaters	

10

Fire extinguishers

All workplaces must have fire-fighting equipment which is easy to access and in good working order. All fire extinguishers are colour-coded to indicate the type of fire they can be used for. Before you use a fire extinguisher, you must read the label to make sure you fully understand what type of fire extinguisher it is and what type of fire it is safe to use on. Using a fire extinguisher is not easy and, unless you are confident that you know how and which one to use, don't try – you could put yourself or others at risk.

Class A
A water extinguisher can be used to put out fires involving paper, coal, textiles and wood

Class B
A foam extinguisher can be used to put out fires involving **flammable** liquids such as grease, oil, petrol and paints (but not cooking oil or grease)

Class C
A carbon dioxide extinguisher can be used to put out fires involving **flammable** gases

Class F
A blanket can be used to put out fires involving cooking oils and fats

Class Electrical
A dry powder extinguisher can be used to put out electrical fires

The Electricity at Work Regulations 1989

This law requires that electrical equipment is safe to use and safely maintained. All electrical appliances must be checked regularly. In a busy salon, this may be every six months. These checks must be carried out either by a qualified electrician or a skilled person who is trained and experienced in the use of that particular appliance, for example, a person employed by the company who supplies the equipment.

All electrical checks must be written in a book that is kept specifically for this reason. The date and signature of the person who carried out the check must be entered along with the reason for the check, for example, whether it was a repair or a just a maintenance check. Information must be given about the nature of the repair or check.

The book must be available for inspection by the health and safety authority.

Your responsibilities at work: electrical appliances

Report to your supervisor immediately: any faulty plugs, frayed wires or loose connections and any flickering or faulty lights.

Do:
- switch off and unplug all machines after use
- check that all equipment trolleys are stable and not on uneven floors
- wind up wires and cables neatly.

Don't:
- touch electrical equipment, plugs or switches with wet hands or place bowls of water nearby
- leave trailing wires
- plug in or use any equipment that has been reported as faulty.

>> **Get up and go!**

Look for pictures on the Internet of three different types of fire-fighting equipment. Cut them out and display them with a brief description of how you would use them and what type of fire they would be used for.

11

Health and safety laws [4]

The Gas Safety (Installation and Use) Regulations 1994

Under these regulations, a workplace must allow gas and HSE inspectors to enter the **premises** in order to disconnect dangerous gas appliances. All gas appliances must be installed, maintained and used safely.

Your responsibilities at work: gas appliances

Report to your supervisor *immediately*:

- any unusual smell
- any regular headaches, nausea (feeling sick) or unexplained tiredness.

The Manual Handling Operations Regulations 1992

The **Health and Safety Executive** introduced the Manual Handling Operations Regulations in 1992 to prevent injury to the muscles and bones of the body. Injury can be caused by:

- wrong lifting methods
- poor posture
- regular and continual strain on the same part of the body
- moving objects by force that may be too heavy.

Posture, lifting and carrying

In the salon, you need to be careful how you lift and carry stock. You also need to take care over the way you sit, whether at reception or while carrying out a treatment – it is important that the chair or couch is the right height for you. To enable your body to change position regularly while working, it is better if you carry out a variety of treatments. In addition, you need to know how to hold tools correctly, and give your hands a chance to rest after a treatment.

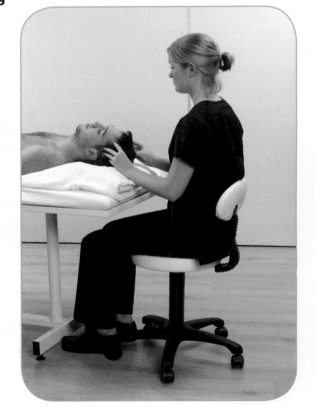

Good posture

Top tips ✓

- If you are unsure about whether you can lift something on your own, always get help.
- If stock needs to be stored on high shelves, make sure you use a safe and stable step ladder – never use a chair.
- Most deliveries are brought to reception. Some are very large and heavy, and will need to be moved elsewhere before they are unpacked. It is very important that large and heavy deliveries are moved carefully to avoid damaging you or the products.

It is a good idea to:

- use height-adjustable couches and stools
- get help when carrying large, heavy or awkward things
- move and stretch your body regularly if you remain in the same position for a long time
- do exercises to keep your hands flexible
- maintain good posture.

Safe lifting method

As a beauty therapist, you will have a lifetime of bending and standing in one position and it is essential that you look after your back. The safe lifting method is shown below; make sure that you follow it.

When picking up a large or heavy item:

- bend at the knee
- use both hands to grasp the box
- use the strength in your legs to help lift the weight
- never bend from the waist, as this could damage your lower back.

Think about the lift. Where is the load to be placed? Do you need help? Are handling aids available?

With your feet close to the load, bend your knees and keep your back straight. Tuck in your chin. Lean slightly forward over the load to get a good grip.

When you are sure of your grip on the load, straighten your legs and lift smoothly. Remember to keep your back straight.

Carry the load close to your body.

Health and safety laws (5)

The Personal Protective Equipment at Work Regulations 1992

These regulations state that staff must have training in the use of equipment, and details the use of protective clothing for safety at work.

Your responsibilities at work: equipment and clothing

- Never use any equipment for which you have not received training.
- Always wear the recommended protective clothing.

The Control of Substances Hazardous to Health Regulations 2002 (COSHH)

This law requires employers to assess the risks from all harmful products and take appropriate precautions. All products that could be harmful must be:

- used safely according to the manufacturer's instructions
- stored safely
- cleaned up safely when spilt
- thrown away safely.

Employers must write down all the products they use, how they are used, stored, cleaned up and thrown away (including cleaning agents). Employers must do this because the products they use could:

- be **flammable**
- be poisonous if swallowed
- cause irritation
- give out strong fumes
- be dangerous if inhaled
- be slippery if spilt.

The simplest way to record information about the different products used by a salon is in a table, which is clear and easy to read. An example is given below.

Get up and go!

Ask your tutor which hazardous substances are used on your course. Ask to look at the list that says how they should be handled.

Top tip ✓

It is very important that the manufacturer's instructions are followed. These are usually shown on the packaging of a product, or on a separate leaflet inside the box.

Product	Hazard	Correct use	Storage	Disposal of waste	Caution
Nail varnish remover	Inhalation of fumes; highly flammable	Replace bottle tops immediately; no smoking or naked flames nearby	Store away from direct heat in a locked cupboard, with lids fully on and bottle upright	Do not dispose of by burning	If spilt, clear up immediately as it can dissolve some plastics such as cushion flooring, and mark trolleys and equipment. If spilt on clothes, minimise the fumes by sponging with water

14

Manufacturer's instructions

All equipment and products used in a salon must be used in line with the manufacturer's instructions and guidelines. If they are used incorrectly they could cause damage, injury or some other danger to the safety of clients and staff. The instructions also cover the disposal and maintenance of products and equipment. Any accidents or injuries that occur when the manufacturer's instructions are not followed would not be covered by the salon's insurance. It is a legal requirement that all instructions are included with all equipment and products, so it is essential that they are followed.

The Health and Safety Regulations (First Aid) 1981

This act tells employers what they must do to help prevent accidents, and how to deal with accidents when they happen. The employer must follow their rules and guidelines.

The main requirements are:

- a suitably stocked first aid box
- an appointed person to take care of first aid arrangements.

What is first aid?

- First aid is the first help given to someone with an injury or who has become ill. It is the treatment given before the person receives professional medical aid.
- First aid includes calling for help or telephoning for an ambulance (if the problem is serious).

First aid does **not** include:

- giving medicines or tablets
- moving a person who has fallen and could possibly have broken bones – his or her injury could be made worse.

The Health and Safety Regulations (First Aid) 1981 state that there should be a member of staff who is trained in first aid. Once this person has been trained, he or she is qualified for three years. After this time, the person will need to re-train.

It is the job of the first aider to try to prevent a casualty from becoming worse before the ambulance or doctor arrives.

Important things to remember when dealing with a casualty are:

- stay calm
- listen to the person and talk quietly to him or her
- be gentle and caring
- move the casualty as little as possible
- keep the person warm with a blanket, but do not allow him or her to get too hot.

Health and safety laws (6)

The first aid box

A first aid kit must be in a proper first aid box. This is a green box with a white cross on the front. A first aid kit must not be kept in any old container, such as a biscuit tin or shoe box.

The first aid box must be kept in a place where all staff can access it easily. It should not be hidden from view and must be labelled clearly.

The first aid box must only contain items that a first aider has been trained to use. It must not contain any medication.

The contents of a first aid box

> **» Get up and go!**
>
> Think about the places where you have worked, or your school/college. Find out the following information:
> - Where are the first aid boxes kept?
> - Do they contain enough of the important first aid items?
> - Are the contents checked regularly so that used items are replaced?

Top tip ✓

Don't place tools in your pockets as many are pointed or sharp and could result in an injury if you fall or bump into someone.

The Environmental Protection Act 1990, Waste Regulations 1992 and Special Waste Regulations 1996

These regulations state that clinical waste must be separated from normal waste and disposed of by licensed incineration. Clinical waste means waste items consisting of human tissue, blood, bodily fluids, swabs, dressings, syringes or needles, and incineration means official and permitted burning.

Your responsibilities at work: clinical waste

- Never dispose of clinical waste in a normal waste bin.

The Local Government (Miscellaneous Provisions) Act 1982

Practitioners who carry out a treatment involving the use of needles or skin piercing must register with their local authority. The workplace **premises** also need to be registered, unless the practitioner is mobile, in which case the registration will be for them only. The cost for this registration differs slightly between different authorities.

After the **premises** or practitioner is registered to carry out the treatments, a local authority inspector will visit to check that the levels of hygiene and safety are satisfactory. Once the checks have been satisfactorily completed, and if the practitioner is qualified, the inspector awards a certificate that allows the following treatments to be carried out:

- acupuncture
- ear and body piercing
- tattooing
- epilation.

Get ahead

Investigate some more health and safety regulations that are not covered here and that you think may be helpful in the future.

Get up and go!

Contact your local council for information on the registration of ear piercing, tattooing and epilation in your area.

? Memory jogger

1 What does COSHH stand for?

2 What does RIDDOR stand for?

3 What is meant by the term 'clinical waste'?

4 How should you bend when picking up a large or heavy item?

5 When did the Health and Safety Executive introduce the Manual Handling Operations Regulations?

  A 1982

  B 1992

  C 1994

  D 2002

6 How would you identify a first aid box?

  A White with a green cross

  B Green all over

  C White all over

  D Green with a white cross

7 List three things to remember when dealing with a casualty.

8 Which treatments must be registered under the Local Government (Miscellaneous Provisions) Act 1982?

9 List four responsibilities for electrical safety while at work.

Workplace policies [1]

Workplace policies and codes of practice

As well as following the Health and Safety at Work Act, your workplace will have its own rules and guidelines for keeping employees and the general public safe. These are called workplace policies or codes of practice.

It is the employer's duty to provide a safe environment for employees. In addition, employees have a duty to co-operate with the workplace policies in order to demonstrate expected standards of behaviour and to make the salon a safer and healthier place to work.

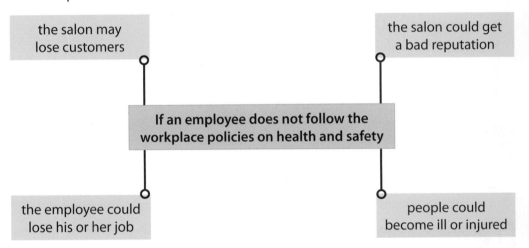

the salon may lose customers

the salon could get a bad reputation

If an employee does not follow the workplace policies on health and safety

the employee could lose his or her job

people could become ill or injured

What are the consequences of not following workplace policies?

Top tip ✓

It is important that you know who to report hazards, risks, accidents, illnesses and injury to. You will need to make sure that you are familiar with these people at the beginning of your work experience and employment.

Get ahead

Design an information sheet that lists all the important people who are responsible for safety in your salon. For example:

1 The name of the first aider(s) and the days on which they work.

2 The name of the salon manager or supervisor who is generally responsible for help and advice in the salon.

3 The following information about the person in charge of health and safety in your salon: their first name and surname; the days/hours he or she works and who is responsible if that person is away; his or her telephone number and/or place of contact.

Get up and go!

If you are doing work experience or have a Saturday job, find out your employer's workplace policies and write them down.

Environmentally friendly practices

When you are ready to throw packaging out, look at the label to see if it can be recycled

Individuals can make changes in their lifestyles to protect the environment, but the biggest changes will happen when companies and manufacturers take up the necessary changes.

For salons and beauty businesses, it is important to use and buy products made from recycled material where possible as this will increase the demand for recycled products and create a good recycling circle. You can do your bit for the environment while at work, school, college and home. Recycle rubbish such as plastic bottles, jars, paper and card.

When it comes to the working environment, being environmentally friendly is even more important as we use more products and materials and produce much more waste. Your working space and practices must promote environmentally friendly practices. This means that:

- you recycle waste – for example, empty product bottles
- you wash bedding and towels at a lower temperature and wash as much as possible at one time
- you are economical with consumables such as cotton wool and couch roll
- you remember to turn off lighting, heating and hot water heaters when they are not being used
- you don't allow taps to run – it is better to turn them on and off regularly.

Buy Fairtrade goods. Fairtrade is all about better prices and decent working conditions, as well as fair terms of trade for farmers and workers in the developing world.

? Memory jogger

1 What does environmentally friendly mean?
2 List three ways that you should be environmentally friendly at work.
3 What does Fairtrade mean?
4 How can you recycle?

» Get up and go!

How many more ways can you think of to be environmentally friendly in the salon environment?

Create an informative poster that you can put on the salon or classroom wall to try to get everyone to think more about being environmentally friendly.

Workplace policies (2)

Salon hygiene

A clean, tidy and organised salon is one that will appeal to clients. However, it is not just important to keep things clean and tidy so that the salon looks good. It is also vital in order to control the spread of bacteria that could be a danger to clients and staff. Bacteria spread very easily though the use of dirty tools, for example. Good salon hygiene is therefore a must.

Passing on infection

Infection can pass from one person to another in two ways: direct contact and indirect contact.

- Direct contact is when an infection passes straight from one person to another. This can occur by touching the skin, sneezing, coughing or breathing.
- Indirect contact is when infection passes from one person to another through an unclean object, such as a towel, a jar of cream, tweezers, a wet floor or dirty equipment and tools. This is called **cross-infection**. Cross-infection is the transfer of germs and bacteria through poor hygiene.

Preventing cross-infection

There are three ways to make sure that the work environment is clean and germ-free.

1 Cleaning

This includes cleaning or washing skin, tools and equipment to promote health by reducing the growth of germs and bacteria. It also removes dust and dirt.

- When cleaning the hands, use liquid soap and paper towels as these are the most hygienic.
- Before any **disinfection** and **sterilisation** (see below), always clean tools and equipment by washing them.
- Chemicals used for cleaning include surface agents (surfactants), alcohols and hypochlorites such as hygiene sprays and gels.

2 Disinfection

Disinfection is a form of cleaning in which surfaces, trolleys and equipment are wiped over with a disinfectant solution.

This reduces the numbers of germs and bacteria to a level that is less harmful to health. Most disinfectant solutions are alcohol- or bleach-based.

For treatments in which the skin must be very clean, such as electrolysis or ear piercing, a disinfectant solution or wipe is used on the skin.

To keep previously sterilised tools (see below) clean during a treatment, place them in a jar of disinfectant solution.

3 Sterilisation

Sterilisation is a cleaning method that kills all germs and bacteria. It is used for tools and equipment. The tools are heated to a very high temperature to kill all germs and bacteria.

>> **Get up and go!**

In your college or salon, look at the list of ingredients on the bottles of the products used for cleaning and disinfecting.

Top tip ✓

Wet hands are not clean hands. It is very important to dry them thoroughly after washing.

However, if the **sterilisation** routine is not thorough, some germs will remain.

There are only two reliable methods of sterilisation:

- dry heat sterilising, which takes place in a hot air oven
- steam sterilising, which takes place in an autoclave.

There are other methods of sterilisation:

- ultraviolet sterilising, which takes place in an ultraviolet cabinet
- heat destruction, which takes place in a bead steriliser.

However, these methods are not always 100 per cent effective at reaching all the surfaces of the tools. In addition, the temperatures can vary in places, so are not always hot enough to kill the germs and bacteria.

Autoclave

Ultraviolet cabinet

Top tip

Disinfection and sterilisation are useless on unclean tools and equipment. Your first step must always be to clean them by washing.

Your responsibilities at work: cutting down the risk of infection

1 Wash and dry your hands before and after each client.

2 Hold sterilised tools by the handle only.

3 Always use clean towels and a protective couch roll for each client.

4 Wipe down surfaces and trolleys with a disinfectant solution regularly.

5 Keep your nails short with no varnish, and tie your hair back neatly.

6 Don't share tools.

7 Remove all jewellery.

8 Use disposable tools where possible.

9 Wear a clean and fresh uniform.

10 Re-sterilise any tools that have been dropped on the floor.

11 Wear a plaster on any cuts or grazes.

12 Replace tops on products straight away.

13 Don't eat and drink in the treatment area.

14 Always use spatulas to remove creams from jars.

15 Never cough, sneeze or blow your nose over a client.

16 Dust and clean the therapist's work area regularly.

17 Don't carry out a treatment if you have a cold or the 'flu.

18 Never treat open cuts, bites or stings.

19 Use sterilised equipment only.

20 Never treat anyone with a contra-indication (you can find more information about this in Units B2, B3 and N1).

Workplace policies (3)

Security and safekeeping

The security of takings, staff, clients and their belongings is important in a salon. No one wants their belongings lost and your employer does not want hard-earned money lost, or worse, stolen. In this section, you will learn about how to protect the workplace, clients and products from theft.

At the salon

A salon owner needs to make sure that the business **premises** are secure. The salon will not be covered on insurance for fire, theft or damage if it is not. It is therefore vital that the correct steps are carried out to secure the building.

When closed:	When open:
All external doors must be locked when the building is empty.	Senior members of staff should bank money regularly.
All windows must be shut and locked at the end of the day.	
Burglar alarms must be turned on.	There should be a secure safe for money that cannot be banked until later in the day.
All money must be banked daily and not left on the premises or in the till.	
The till must be emptied at the end of the day and left open.	There should be an electronic till, which is used by one or two members of staff only.
A security nightlight should be installed, to deter burglars.	
A trustworthy person, either a member of staff or a neighbour, should be given a spare key in case of emergency; the person's name and address should be given to the police.	All visitors must be checked in at reception.

Health and Safety at Work Act 1974

Within this act it states that all employers must provide a safe system of cash handling. For example, if an employee is sent to the bank to pay money in alone and is then robbed or mugged, the employer could be prosecuted.

Staff and clients

To avoid loss, theft or damage of goods and valuables that belong to staff and clients, lockers should be provided for valuables and handbags. Staff should avoid bringing valuables or large sums of money to work and clients should keep their handbags and valuables with them at all times, unless client lockers are available in the salon. Clients should themselves place jewellery or valuables in their handbag, or keep such items in full view during a treatment.

Stock

To protect stock against theft, the stock cupboard should remain locked and the key kept in a safe place, preferably in the office. One or two senior members of staff should be responsible for giving out stock for treatments and refilling of products, and products for retail should be kept in full view of the reception desk in a locked display cabinet. The key for the cabinet should be placed on a hook behind the reception

Top tip

As a trainee, it is not your responsibility to take money to the bank for paying in or to handle large amounts of money.

desk, where it cannot be seen or reached by visitors. If a locked cabinet is not available for displaying products, the empty boxes should be put on display and the products kept in the locked stock cupboard. Finally, you should carry out weekly stock checks to make sure that the amounts of stock match with what should be there.

Insurance

Employer's Liability (Compulsory Insurance) Act 1969

This insurance is compulsory for employers and business owners. All employees, clients and visitors to the salon must be covered under this insurance in case they injure themselves or catch a disease at work. The certificate of insurance must be displayed in the workplace for all to see. It will include the following details:

- the name of the business and owner
- the type of business
- the start date and end date of the insurance
- the name of the insurance company.

Your employer may also have professional indemnity insurance. This covers claims against employees if they cause injury or damage to a client or client's property through their irresponsible actions and behaviour. (If an employee does not take out this insurance, they must make sure that they are fully covered on the employer's liability insurance.)

If the salon building is rented or leased the property owner is responsible for insuring it against fire or damage. However, if the building is owned by the salon, the salon owner will need to take out buildings insurance. Finally, the contents of the business will need to be insured against accidental damage, fire or theft. Contents insurance covers items such as tools, equipment, furniture, products and valuables, although this insurance will not cover damage caused through **negligence** or natural wear and tear.

> ## ≫ Get up and go!
>
> Check out how many insurance liability certificates you can see in different shops, offices and businesses that you go into. Every business, including beauty salons, must have these displayed so that people can see them. How many are you able to see?

> ## ? Memory jogger
>
> 1 Who or what does employer's liability insurance protect?
>   A Employers
>   B Staff and visitors
>   C Buildings
>   D Business contents
> 2 What is professional indemnity insurance?
> 3 What insurance is compulsory for employers and business owners?

Personal presentation and behaviour

A high standard of presentation and hygiene at work is necessary in order to follow the salon guidelines and communicate the salon's image as a clean and professional place of business. It will also give clients a good impression of you, as well as making you feel more confident.

Personal hygiene

You must always take care to ensure good personal hygiene at work.

Your personal presentation is very important

Action	How it improves personal hygiene
Bath or shower daily	To remove stale sweat, which will begin to smell as bacteria grows in it
Use an underarm anti-perspirant or deodorant daily	To keep you smelling fresh and to cut down on sweating
Step up your mouth hygiene! Look after your teeth and gums: ■ clean your teeth twice daily ■ floss daily ■ rinse with a mouthwash while at work	Clean teeth and gums mean fresh breath. If you continue to have a mouth odour problem, you could have a build-up of old food around your teeth and gums A mouthwash will help to keep your mouth fresh and stop bacteria from growing in your mouth
Wear a clean, ironed uniform	Uniforms can easily become dirty and absorb smells in the environment, including smells from other people and body odour
Have short, neat nails with no varnish	Dirt, germs and bacteria build up under long nails. Varnish-free nails look cleaner and fresher than painted ones. Some clients can be sensitive to the ingredients in nail varnish
Wash your hands with soap and dry them thoroughly after every visit to the toilet	If you do not wash and dry your hands thoroughly, you may pass many bacteria and germs to others when you carry out a treatment
Never eat in the treatment area	Eating in the treatment area causes the spread of bacteria and will encourage the presence of insects and disease-spreading flies
Remove jewellery when carrying out a treatment	Bacteria can build up under rings

Personal conduct

Conducting yourself positively and behaving in the right way is something that you will need to do throughout your working life. Positive behaviour ranges from demonstrating good body language and good posture, to fair treatment and respect of others along with a willingness to learn.

Your salon will have policies for behaviour and good conduct and these must be followed at all times, otherwise you could risk your job or work experience placement. Salons, as with all public places, must be a non-smoking environment, but remember that even if staff have a cigarette outside during a break, the smell remains on their clothes and breath and can be smelt by clients during their treatment. An alcohol- and drug-free workplace is also essential. Any member of staff under the influence of drugs or alcohol cannot use equipment and products safely and could put others at risk. If clients are under the influence of drugs or alcohol, they will be asked to leave by the supervisor or relevant person.

 Salon life

Karen was going to do her work experience at Vitality and Vitesse. Although she thought the salon looked great, Lindy, her manager, was strict and seemed obsessed with the appearance of her staff when she interviewed Karen.

Karen was only there for two weeks so didn't have the usual staff uniform, but was allowed to wear black trousers and a black t-shirt and flat shoes. On her first day, Lindy looked over Karen's workwear and told her that her trousers were too long and frayed at the edges, her t-shirt was too short and showed off her tummy and pierced navel and that her peep-toe shoes were too high. Karen said that this was all she had at home and her mum couldn't afford to buy her new clothes and shoes just for the two weeks. Lindy explained that she had made the dress code very clear at the interview. Karen then had to work in the laundry room on her first day and Lindy said that she would arrange a spare uniform for the following day.

Karen washed, tumbled and ironed her way throughout the day as well as fetching and carrying up and down the stairs for the therapists. At 12 o'clock Janice, the apprentice, dropped a pair of nail scissors and they fell right on Karen's toes poking out from her peep-toe shoes. Later she was asked to carry some fresh towels up to the treatment rooms with Suki but on the way up the stairs, Suki trod on her long, frayed trousers and Karen fell over. Luckily, she wasn't badly hurt, just shaken up, and after a cup of tea she went back to ironing some duvet covers for the couches. She didn't concentrate, though, and leant on the iron, which burnt her bare tummy. That really was the last straw for Karen and she burst out crying and stormed out of the salon.

Why is it important to present yourself properly?

What could happen if you try to bend the rules about dress code and behaviour?

 Get ahead

Research your workplace's code of conduct. Why do you think it has each rule? What would be the consequences of not following the rules?

? Memory jogger

1 Why are good personal presentation and conduct important at work?

2 Why should you remove jewellery before carrying out a treatment?

Getting ready for assessment

What you must cover during your practical assessments

Safe, healthy and hygienic working practices should be something that you demonstrate throughout all of your practical treatments. It should not be something that you follow just to pass an assessment. For example, when you are being assessed carrying out a facial you will be able to cover G20 performance criteria and your assessor will be able to sign you off for different areas each time.

Carrying out a practical treatment using unhygienic tools, or without carrying out a risk assessment of your work area to avoid accidents happening, will mean that you are not safe to do a treatment and therefore could mean that you do not pass your assessment.

What you must know

In order to pass this unit you will need to know about information and regulations that are relevant to health and safety. You will gather evidence on this during classwork and further study and will probably file it in a portfolio of evidence. This evidence will also be signed off in your candidate log book, which you will be given by your assessor. This will be an official record to show that you have covered what you need to.

Top tips ☑

- Before using any products or equipment read the manufacturer's instructions and follow any previous instructions given to you by your assessor.
- Keep a look out for any unsafe practices.
- Report any hazards to your assessor immediately.

 Salon life

Maz had been working at the Green Rooms for three weeks and although she enjoyed it she found it a nuisance that there were so many rules and regulations that the staff had to follow. She felt it really wasn't necessary; the list of rules seemed endless, and she kept getting into trouble for the slightest thing. For example, yesterday she threw out some empty product bottles and was told that they could be used again. The day before she got told off for using too much cotton wool and tissue, and the day before that she left some bottle tops off the nail varnishes and her manager got really cross. The previous week she felt really cold but had forgotten her work cardigan, so shut the windows and turned off the air conditioning – yes, you can guess, she got in trouble for that as well.

What are the things that Maz did wrong and why do you think they were wrong?

What could happen if everyone constantly did the things that Maz had done?

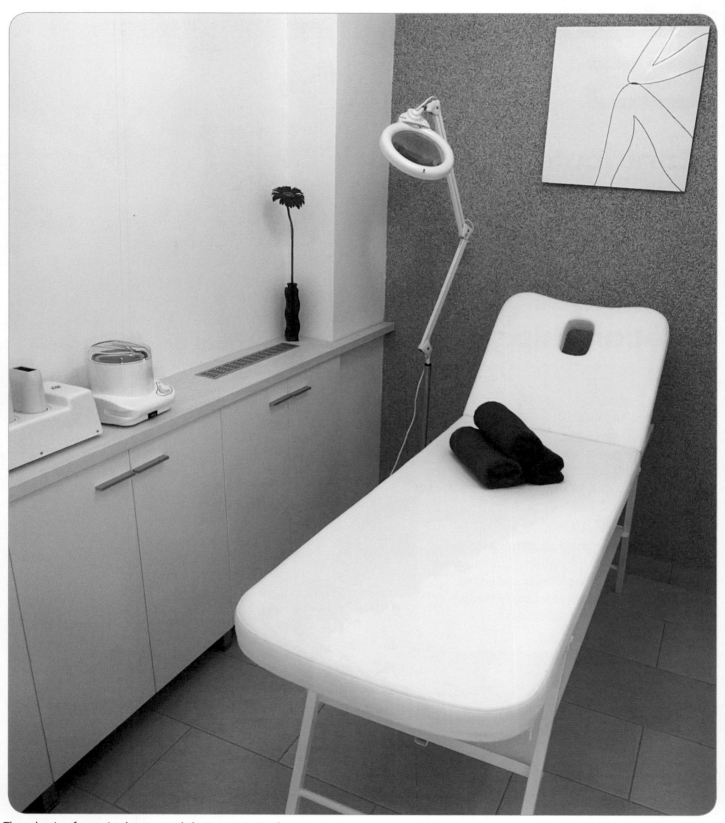

The salon is a fantastic place to work, but you must make
sure that you follow health and safety regulations

UNIT G3

Contribute to the development of effective working relationships

During your career in beauty therapy you will need to form and maintain good working relationships with clients and colleagues. If positive working relationships are not maintained, this could result in an unhappy atmosphere at work, lack of trust and a drop in clientele.

Effective working relationships will help you to enjoy your work, and if all members of the team work together the running of a business is like finding all of the pieces of the jigsaw puzzle. If one piece falls apart many things within the business will suffer or fail.

In this unit you will learn how to:

- Develop effective working relationships with clients
- Develop effective working relationships with colleagues
- Develop yourself within your job role

Here are some key terms you will meet in this unit:

Scripts –
set lists of words to use

Aggression –
anger, annoyance or loss of temper

Commission –
a small percentage of the price of a product that is given to the person who sells it

Target –
aim, ambition, purpose

Overtime –
extra work beyond your normal working hours

Tactless remarks –
remarks made without any thought or consideration as to how they will annoy or upset the person who hears them

Adapt –
change in order to meet different needs

Anticipate –
expect, wait for

Resentment –
dislike, bitterness or anger

Prioritising –
putting the most important things first

Grievance –
cause to complain

Personal development plan –
a plan of how you will develop your job role and career

Promotion –
moving up to a more senior job

Trade journals –
magazines for the industry

Confidence –
when you have a positive feeling or opinion about someone or something

Develop effective working relationships with clients [1]

A salon builds its reputation on how satisfied clients and visitors are. If clients leave the salon unhappy, angry and upset, the word soon spreads to other people and bookings for treatments and services will fall. This means that building effective working relationships with your clients is vital to the successful running of the business. Being a therapist can be very much like being an actress at times; even when you aren't feeling very happy yourself you must not let this show. The client is spending money to feel good and you will be expected to do your best to help their visit go well. As you spend your working day attending to and treating clients, being able to develop good relationships with them will also help to increase the enjoyment that you get from your work.

Appearance and hygiene

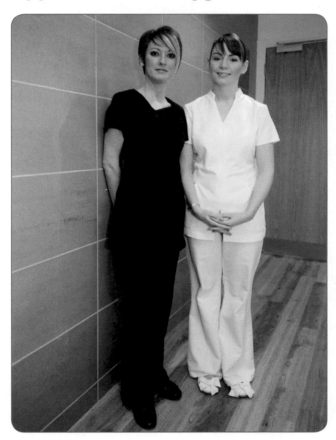

You must always look professional

How you look and behave will obviously affect how your clients feel about their experience in your salon. Looking professional and behaving professionally will help to give your clients **confidence** in you.

Your salon will have rules about appearance and you will be told how you must present yourself and, whether you think it is fashionable or not, you must follow what you are told. You must make sure that you are freshly showered each day and that you have clean, fresh breath.

Top tip ✓

If clients are unhappy and don't re-book, it will eventually have a knock-on effect for jobs.
No clients = no jobs.

Uniform

All salons have their own style and how they want their staff to look. Some salons prefer white whereas others prefer black or colour. The uniforms could be dresses, tunics and skirts, or tunics and trousers.

Whatever you are expected to wear as part of the salon's look, it must be clean, ironed and hemmed and without any buttons missing or broken zips. The smallest dip in standards of appearance will be noticed by your supervisor and the clients and you would be letting yourself down as well as them. Shoes must usually be low heeled and enclosed for health and safety reasons.

The other reason why uniform is worn is for protection while you work. This comes under the Personal Protective Equipment at Work Regulations, which was covered on page 14.

Hair

Hair must usually be tied up, making sure there is no loose hair around your face and neck that could dangle on a client's skin when doing a treatment. It must also be very clean and most definitely not smell of smoke.

Jewellery

Small earrings that don't hang are acceptable, as well as a watch, but otherwise all other jewellery should be removed.

Behaviour

You must act in a professional manner at all times when in the salon. Having the right attitude is important no matter who you are working with, whether it is your supervisor, other colleagues or clients.

Your employer will have certain standards for behaviour, and there may be a list of rules. Make sure that you are aware of them all and that you follow them. Failing to follow rules could mean that you lose your job, but making sure that you follow your salon's standards will help you to develop effective relationships at work, as well as making sure that you, your clients and your colleagues remain as safe as possible at all times.

Always follow these basic rules.

- Talk properly without use of slang.
- Turn off mobile phones and don't text friends.
- Don't gossip or chat during work hours.
- Maintain good posture, as slouching around looks as though you don't care.
- Don't shout across a room – go over and talk quietly instead.
- Don't smoke on the premises or in view of clients outside the building.
- Don't eat or drink except in the staff room.

 Get up and go!

Record three examples of people on the telephone, either making appointments or answering enquiries (you could do this on your mobile phone). Then let the rest of the class hear and ask them to decide who they think sounds the best and the most professional. Ask for ideas as to how the others could be improved.

Develop effective working relationships with clients (2)

Communication

The key to all good relationships, whether personal, business or work relationships, is effective communication. There are many different forms of communication, but all are built on our ability to pass on information, feelings and understanding through speaking, writing or body language.

Different methods of communication include:

- Oral communication – speaking to another person. This includes speaking by telephone or face-to-face conversations.
- Written communication – for example, letters, memos, faxes, text messages and email.
- Body language – for example nodding, smiling and making eye contact.
- Images – communicating information through adverts, posters, magazines and brochures.

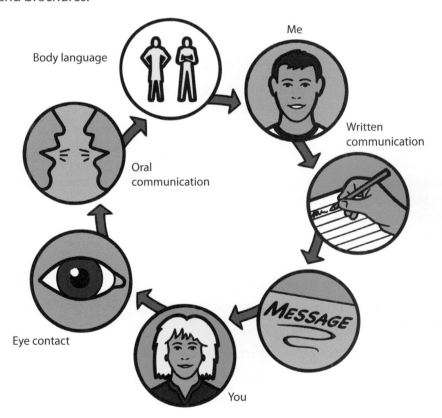

Methods of communication

Positive and negative communication

As we have seen, communication does not just mean what you say out loud. You also communicate with people through the way in which you use words and your body language. It is important that all of the messages that you communicate are positive ones.

All of your messages should be positive

Sometimes, if you are not feeling great, it can be hard to make sure that you use only positive methods of communication. However, no matter how you are feeling, the use of negative methods will not be a successful way to get your message or point across.

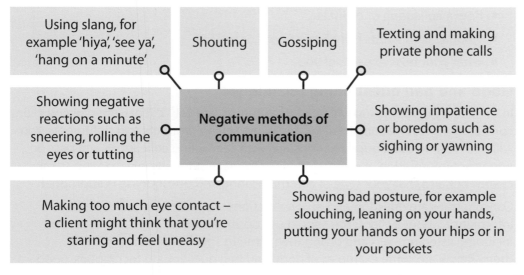

Negative methods of communication are not a good way to express yourself

Always pay attention to your body language as you might communicate a negative message to a client or colleague, for example that you are bored, without really meaning to. These negative methods are all barriers to communication and should never be used at work. Think about how you would react if someone used these negative methods with you.

In order to show a good image of yourself and the salon to clients, and to maintain good relationships with your colleagues, you must communicate clearly, politely and confidently. Clients need to feel that they can trust you and that you will maintain their confidentiality.

Develop effective working relationships with clients (3)

Questioning and listening skills

Communicating is not just about getting your own message across – it is about understanding, interpreting and reacting to messages that other people might be giving you, and also about asking questions.

Good questioning skills will help you to find out about:

- job roles and responsibilities
- a person's personality
- how a client or colleague may be feeling.

Quite often people ask questions without really listening to the answer. This is not a good way to communicate and you could miss valuable information such as:

- how a colleague or client is
- what a client wants from a treatment or service
- what your boss expects of you.

Good and bad questioning techniques

In the beauty industry, you will need to communicate with clients when giving client consultations, advice and aftercare, and when selling products and treatments. You will also need to build good relationships with clients and colleagues and pass on important information. You therefore need to make sure not only that you speak clearly, but also that your style of communicating and questioning is appropriate.

Consultations are question-and-answer sessions that are designed to find out information about a client. You should use positive methods of communication including listening skills and giving them time to speak before interrupting them. Below are some examples of good and bad questioning techniques: good questioning uses open questions that allow a full answer, whereas bad questioning techniques use closed questions that result in a 'Yes' or 'No' answer.

- Good: 'Tell me about your skin care routine at home.'
- Bad: 'Do you cleanse, tone and moisturise at home?'

Recognising a client's moods

Knowing when a client is happy, annoyed or confused is important. If you are unable to recognise different moods or mood changes in a client you will have no idea what is wrong with them and how you might put it right.

Here are some typical signals that may tell you a client is not happy.

- Huffing – may suggest she is fed up with with being kept waiting.
- Tutting – may suggest that she is annoyed.
- A grumpy expression – could mean she is not enjoying her treatment.
- Tapping her fingers on a surface – may suggest that you are running late.

» Get up and go!

Think of some positive questions that could be used during a consultation and then think of an opposite, negative one for each to demonstrate the difference.

» Get up and go!

In pairs, one of you should imagine that you are unhappy with a service and give non-oral signs to suggest that you are fed up. Your partner should watch carefully and read your body language.

34

The client's facial expression can also tell you if they are confused. Look out for:

- one eyebrow higher than the other
- a wrinkled nose and crease between the eyebrows
- a raised corner of the mouth.

Another sign may be that they keep asking you to explain the same thing or question you about the same thing, which suggests that they have not received a good enough answer or an answer that is easy to understand.

Rules and procedures

Salon businesses usually have set communication methods and procedures that they expect employees to follow. Some even have set **scripts** that employees need to follow. These may include how to answer the phone, re-book appointments and carry out client consultations.

It is very important that you follow these procedures because they are part of the business's identity and ensure that all staff are following a set of guidelines for communicating with clients, visitors and each other.

Client care

A salon builds its reputation on how satisfied clients are. Many salons will have guidelines for client care and these may include some of the following procedures.

Handling client belongings

When a client undresses or removes jewellery, let her see where you are putting it for safekeeping so that she knows where it is. Fold her clothes with care or hang them up and place her jewellery in a bowl that she can see easily. It is better to give it to the client for safekeeping, though. At the end of the treatment, pass her the clothes and the bowl of jewellery stating what you are doing so that there is no confusion.

Referring client concerns

If at any time your client is worried or has a question that you are unable to answer, you must refer this promptly to a senior member of staff.

Maintaining client comfort and care

Pay attention to client comfort and care before, during and after their treatment. Before the treatment:

- greet them and collect them from reception
- use positive communication and body language.

During the treatment:

- check that they are warm, comfortable and relaxed
- maintain positive communication.

After the treatment:

- check their satisfaction with the treatment
- offer to help them with their coat and belongings
- offer to book their next appointment
- take them back to reception and say goodbye.

> **? Memory jogger**
>
> 1 List three types of positive communication.
> 2 List three types of negative communication.
> 3 What is the difference between an open and a closed question?

Develop effective working relationships with colleagues (1)

Working with other people in a salon is not always easy. It can be necessary for very different personalities to work together in a small environment. Being helpful and supportive while making a positive contribution to the team effort will help you to achieve success with both your workmates and your manager.

You won't necessarily always have great relationships with your colleagues at work. You will need to accept that everyone you work with is different. You are not expected to like all your colleagues, no matter how hard you may try, but you must be able to get along with them. This means that you must respect each other's differences and build good working relationships.

Factors contributing to good working relationships

Teamwork

Teamwork simply means working with others or working together to reach a common goal. At work, staff often work in teams to carry out roles and responsibilities: two heads can often be better than one. As a beauty therapist assistant, assisting other therapists and learning from them are key to your role.

Teamwork is about thinking how you can support the business and colleagues.

- Make yourself useful – keep yourself busy.
- Be available – don't disappear into the staffroom at every opportunity.
- Be ready and willing to assist.
- Try to **anticipate** needs of colleagues and clients, for example by preparing work areas, tools and equipment and products before they have to ask.
- Always wear a smile and be ready to help.

What you need to do when working with colleagues

Top tips ✓

- A successful business employs reliable and hard-working staff who work well together as a team.
- Teamwork is about give and take.

Top tips

- Teamwork also means sharing work – not necessarily doing the same job, but sharing workloads relating to common tasks.
- There are always jobs to do that are less popular than others, or times when staff are needed to do **overtime**. Don't let it always be the same people who put in the extra effort. If that person is always you, you should be prepared to say 'no' and suggest a fairer system. If you always sneak off when jobs need doing, ask yourself, 'Am I being fair?'

 Salon life

Since Debbie and Tracey started work at the Serene Spa, they found it difficult to agree on anything. Debbie found Tracey very bossy, even though they were both assistant therapists.

It all came to a head on Saturday afternoon. The day had been very busy and very long, and Debbie was sick of Tracey ordering her about. 'Tidy this up', 'Have you cut up the cotton wool?', 'Go and work on reception', 'Change the couch roll' – the list was endless. Who did she think she was?

When Tracey told Debbie to sweep the reception area Debbie snapped and started shouting at her and told her she was sick of her being so bossy and then told her to sweep up herself! The reception area went deathly quiet and the clients waiting for treatments looked shocked and uncomfortable. Trish, the salon manager, ordered Debbie into the office.

Who was in the wrong – Debbie or Tracey?

What could have been done to stop the situation getting this bad?

What could Debbie have done instead of losing her temper?

 Get ahead

Find out the differences between aggressive, assertive and passive behaviour in the workplace. Then observe your colleagues or classmates while they are working in a practical session and make notes on whether you think each of them demonstrate aggressive, assertive or passive behaviour and the reasons why.

Present this information as a PowerPoint presentation and deliver your findings to the group with opportunity for discussion afterwards.

Develop effective working relationships with colleagues (2)

Communicating with colleagues

Working effectively with your colleagues will include exchanging different types of information with them and using positive methods of communication. This is just as important when you are working with colleagues as it is when you are working with clients.

Some subjects might be difficult to bring up, such as if you need to tell a colleague that you are unhappy about something they have done or if you need to report a problem to your manager/supervisor, but this means that you need to take even more care to communicate positively.

To work successfully as part of a team you need to listen to other people's views even though you may not agree with them. When you want to put an important point across, you should speak in a calm voice without showing **aggression**. There is more chance that you will be taken seriously and listened to if you don't get angry or lose your temper. Making **tactless remarks** could hurt or offend people. Remember, there is always room for different views and opinions.

It is important to report any information you have been given to the appropriate person straight away, or if this is not possible a note should be left for them. If a colleague needs to know something so that they can carry out their job or deal with a client properly, this information must not be left until later as it could affect how the salon runs.

Top tip

To run successfully, a salon relies on timely reporting of information.

Respect

You need to have respect for your colleagues to ensure good staff relations. Problems that come up should be discussed immediately. If they are not talked about, **resentment** may build up and this will lead to a bad atmosphere that will spill over into your work. This negative atmosphere may be picked up by clients and other staff members, affecting the salon as a whole.

It is also a good idea to build relationships with other members of staff by checking anything with them that may affect them or their work. If you don't, this could lead to bad feeling and cause conflict. Try to be fair to others and respect their views, methods and belongings.

A negative atmosphere will affect the salon as a whole

Top tips

- Try to get on with all of your colleagues.
- Stay calm and try not to lose your temper.
- Respect the fact that not everyone thinks in the same way that you do.
- Try some relaxation techniques to calm you down when you need to.
- Treat people with respect and in the way that you would wish to be treated.
- Don't bring your arguments to work.
- Be supportive of each other's ideas and career plans.

Get up and go!

Write a short script in pairs that demonstrates good and bad examples of working relationships and perform this as a role play to the rest of the group.

Reporting difficulties in working with others

At some point in your career you will have difficulties with other colleagues. This could be as simple as a disagreement, but could go from bad to worse if you do not refer problems to a senior member of staff. It is not about telling tales but instead it is about trying to work out any difficulties that you have so that you stay professional and keep the workplace a calm and happy place to work in.

Get up and go!

Describe the 'ideal' working colleague using a spidergram (there is an example of a spidergram on page 36).

Summary

As a team we should:

- support one another
- watch out for each other
- work well with each other
- communicate well with each other.

Memory jogger

1 Why is it important to communicate well with colleagues?

2 What could happen if the staff in a salon didn't work as a team?

3 Why must you treat your colleagues with respect?

Develop yourself within your job role (1)

As a Level 1 student you are at the beginning of an exciting career in beauty therapy. It is really important that from the start of your employment you are clear about what your role involves, what your salon expects of you and what your limits of authority are so that you know how to do your job properly. You also need to consider the importance of how to develop yourself within your role so that you can move on from Level 1 to the next step in your beauty therapy career.

Finding out about your job

As discussed in Unit G20 Make sure your own actions reduce risks to health and safety, the legal requirements that salons have play a large part in their success and reputation. As well as this all salons have their own rules and regulations.

Contract of employment

When you get a job you will have a contract of employment. This will cover all sorts of things such as:

- hours you work
- holidays per year
- pension schemes
- disciplinary and **grievance** procedures
- sick pay
- your job role and responsibilities.

Induction

Get ahead

Imagine that you are a salon reception manager.

What things would you cover in your reception induction for new staff?

How would you make sure that your induction had worked?

In addition to receiving your contract of employment, you will also have an induction when you first start a new job or attend work experience. This can be carried out on a one-to-one basis or, if a few new employees are starting at the same time, it may be carried out in a group.

This induction will cover the important information that you need to know about your job, the roles you have and your responsibilities. For example:

- who you report to
- what you must do each day
- health and safety
- members of the staff
- the time you start and finish work
- standards of appearance and behaviour.

Without an induction you would not know what you can and cannot do, what to do if there was an emergency and who you will be working with. It is a large part of your role as a beauty therapy assistant to find out about your salon's requirements and what they will expect of you.

As well as this you will be expected to keep up to date with things about your job. New methods, rules and procedures may be introduced or improvements made to ones already in place. See the information on continuous professional development on page 46 for advice on how to make sure you keep up to date with new developments in the beauty therapy industry.

Attendance and punctuality

Employers expect their staff to have a good attendance record. Staff who take lots of time off can cause difficulties for the business and their colleagues. Not only will the business be short staffed and unable to book as many clients during that time, but the other employees will have to work harder to make up for the person who is away, which puts extra pressure on them at work.

Everyone is ill at some point and this cannot be helped, but it is the people who are continually absent from work that can cause problems for others.

Just as frustrating is the employee who is always late. This means that the day starts badly, things are not prepared, colleagues have to cover until the person eventually arrives and clients can be kept waiting.

Seeking permission

A beauty therapy assistant is the first rung on a ladder to a career in the beauty industry and this means that you will always need to get permission from your supervisor before doing anything more than what you have been told to do. This is to make sure that you, your colleagues and your clients stay safe. Make sure that you are aware of your limits of authority and that you do not overstep them.

Reporting difficulties

A range of difficulties may come up during your working day. These could include:

- problems with another colleague
- too much work to do and not enough time
- not understanding instructions and needing further help
- a mistake that you have made.

It is important to report any difficulty that you are unable to deal with to someone more senior, no matter how small it is, as small problems can become large ones if left.

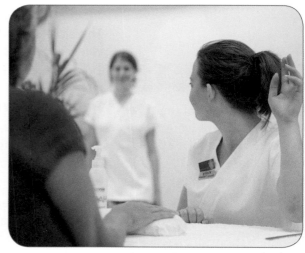

Make sure that you report any difficulties you come across

Salon grievance and appeals procedures

Each salon should have a **grievance** and appeals procedure. This may be a simple document that includes information on things such as what to do if you feel that you are being treated unfairly, for example:

- workplace bullying
- being expected to work outside your normal working hours constantly
- being expected to do jobs that you are not qualified to do
- disagreements with others that cannot be sorted out
- working conditions.

It is important that you know about the salon's staffing structure so that you know who is responsible for what and who you need to ask or discuss things with. If you felt that you were being treated unfairly, you should report this to your named supervisor.

 Get ahead

Research on the Internet and find out more about grievance and appeals procedures in the workplace.

Develop yourself within your job role (2)

Procedures and targets

For the salon to be successful, the business and the staff need set procedures and **targets**. Having manageable targets gives everyone something to aim for, especially when a reward is offered if targets are met. A good beauty business recognises this and offers its staff extras on top of their wages if they meet targets and prove themselves to be valuable employees.

Business development targets

Salon businesses set targets for their staff to achieve. This is because they need them to boost the takings and success of the business. Quite often the salon will give their staff an incentive to meet the targets. Targets could be selling products, promoting new treatments or having a busy column.

An incentive could be a **commission** on sales and treatments. This means that staff receive a small percentage of the sales and treatments over and above their normal wages. A typical method might be 10 per cent of the money taken from sales.

Therefore, if a therapist earns £150 per week and sells £50 worth of products in a week, her wages would work out at:

£150 + 10% of £50 (£5) = £155.

Personal development targets

Personal effectiveness in your work role involves aiming all the time to improve your performance. It is based on lots of different things, such as how successfully you communicate, your willingness to do the job, your attitude and how supportive you are to others.

Your personal performance can be developed as you learn a new job and gain new skills. An important framework for this is a **personal development plan**. Creating a personal development plan involves setting personal **targets** related to your training and career. These are usually based around your performance at work, and your future career aims and plans, such as training and **promotion**.

Setting targets related to these will involve identifying your strengths and weaknesses. Being aware of these will help you to focus on building on what you are good at and improving on what you are not so good at.

Weaknesses are often due to a lack of knowledge and experience and can often be improved with training and experience. For example, you may think that your reception skills are weak, but this may be because you lack **confidence** with clients and experience at the tasks involved in running a reception. With practice and training your confidence will grow and your weaknesses can eventually become your strengths.

Get ahead ⬆

Work out what each of the following therapists would take home in pay at the end of a week, based on a 10 per cent **commisssion** rate:

- If Claire earns £165 and sells £75 worth of products, how much will her wages be?

- If Matt earns £100 as an apprentice and sells £160 worth of products, how much will his wages be?

Use the table below as a fun way of gaining a clearer picture of the type of person you are. Identify the qualities you think you have from those listed in the table below, and give an example of how you show each quality.

≫ Get up and go!

Quality	Personal example	Quality	Personal example
Punctual		Often late	
A good listener		Doesn't pay attention to others or interrupts	
Uncompetitive		Competitive	
Laid back, never feels rushed		Always in a rush	
Patient, particularly with waiting		Impatient, hates to wait	
Concentrates on one thing at a time – unable to multi-task		Able to multi-task, often taking on too many things	
Slow, deliberate talker		Exuberant, fast talker	
Able to motivate self without the need for praise		Needs constant praise and recognition	
Slow-paced		Does everything at a fast pace, even walking, eating and talking	
Relaxed and easy-going		Tense and stressed	
Expresses feelings		Hides feelings	
Lots of outside interests		Few interests – hard to find the time or energy	
Unambitious		Ambitious, driven	

Once you have identified your strengths and weaknesses in terms of your work, you need to discuss these with your tutor or supervisor at work, and have them agreed. You then need to set some targets and deadlines for achieving those targets and record these, with your supervisor, on your **personal development plan**. It is important that your targets are realistic.

Continually using your personal development plan and updating it as necessary will provide your learning at work with a structure. Working towards meeting your personal targets will help you to grow as a valuable employee and will motivate you to progress on to the next step in your career.

Here are some possible targets that you might set yourself:

- short term (three months) – to pass ten assessments
- medium term (nine months) – to pass all assessments and gain the NVQ Level 1 Beauty Therapy
- long term (three years) – to gain Level 2 or Level 3 Beauty Therapy.

Meeting your targets has a number of positive benefits to you. These include respect from others, a sense of satisfaction, promotion and wage improvement.

? Memory jogger

1 How can setting targets help you?

2 When you receive an amount of extra money in your wages from salon sales and treatments, this is called:

C An incentive

D Commission

E Personal development

F A percentage

Develop yourself within your job role (3)

Reviews and feedback

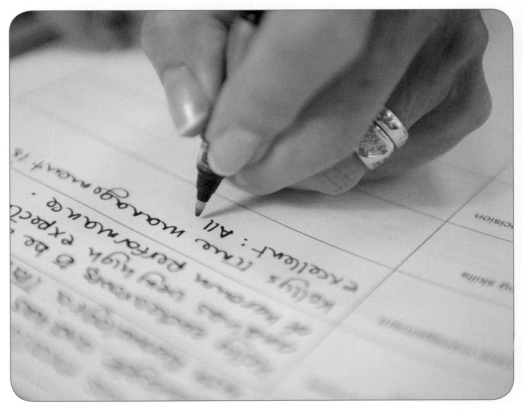

An appraisal form

An important part of improving your performance and developing yourself within your job role is reviewing your progress on a regular basis, both by yourself, with your colleagues and with your employer or tutor. Part of working with others is being able to accept feedback and reviews. Your supervisor will give you feedback on your work regularly. This is not meant to be critical, but is a positive process aimed at improving your performance and helping you to meet your targets. You will need to listen and not take offence.

As well as regular feedback during your career, you will have official reviews called appraisals. These are a formal opportunity for you and your boss to discuss your progress and how you both think you are doing, and for you both to assess whether or not you have met your targets. Did you meet all of your targets within the time scale you set? If not, why not? What did you do well? Are there any areas where you had particular difficulties or where you need more specific training?

You will be able to use the feedback from your appraisal, both on your achievements and on the areas that you need to develop, to set yourself new targets for your future **personal development plan** and to help you progress to the next step in your career.

Taking personal responsibility for your own development

Remember that how well you do at work and how fast you progress is largely down to you. It is important to take responsibility for your own development. If you feel that you have not been given clear enough instructions when you have been asked to do a task, make sure that you ask the relevant person as soon as possible. If you don't ask, you might not be told. If you find a part of your work difficult, ask your supervisor to help you. Remember they all started off as assistants and trainees too.

If you are given opportunities to learn, take advantage of them. Take part as actively as possible in all of the training and development activities you have the chance to be involved in, and take an active role in salon activities. Watch your more senior colleagues perform technical treatments and learn from them.

Managing your time

So that you can manage your time successfully, you need to know what your goals are so that you can plan your time. For example, if your boss has given you a list of jobs to do, you will need to work out how much time you have got to do them in so that you can decide which ones are the most important. This is called **prioritising**.

If you don't learn to manage your time, you may not get the things done that you need to and could become stressed. Things that you will need to time-manage in the salon include:

- preparing the work area for the next client
- cleaning up the work area before the next client is due
- following senior therapists' instructions and making sure you carry them out in time
- arriving for work on time.

Time management is also important in your personal life as this can affect how punctual you are at work. Things that you need to time-manage outside of work include:

- job tasks
- homework
- jobs around the house
- time for friends
- time for relaxing.

Time management should work for you and should have some flexibility so that you can alter or change your priorities if you need to.

 Top tip

As a beauty therapist, you should aim to be hard-working and reliable. This means that you work to the best of your abilities and don't need constant supervision. Flexibility is also a great advantage. Try to **adapt** to changing circumstances and situations without complaining.

Develop yourself within your job role [4]

Continuous professional development (CPD)

It is not enough to gain a qualification in beauty therapy as techniques, products and skills are changing and improving all of the time, especially with the introduction of new things. Therefore, you must continually try to improve by going on training courses, attending exhibitions, reading **trade journals** and sharing ideas and tips with other therapists.

After you have qualified as a therapist

Spend every possible moment developing your knowledge and practising your skills. Don't relax just because you have a qualification. Read every book, magazine and trade journal you can lay your hands on to get the latest beauty buzz word on everyone's lips.

Attend trade shows, exhibitions and workshops for professional development. Never think you know it all just because you have qualified.

Join professional organisations to keep you informed about new developments and in contact with other therapists that you can share knowledge, advice and good practice with.

Trade journals

The **trade journals** listed below are written especially for everyone involved in the health and beauty industry and are a good source of professional information. The journals are essential reading for keeping up to date with treatment techniques, new products, cosmetic trends, trade events and celebrity personalities influencing the trade. Journals include:

- *Guild News*
- *Health and Beauty Salon*
- *International Therapist*
- *Professional Beauty*
- *Professional Nails*
- *Salon Today*
- *Tanning World*
- *Today's Therapist*.

Top tip

Visit the Salon International and Professional Beauty websites to find about these exhibitions. You can access the websites by going to www.pearsonhotlinks.co.uk and searching for this title.

Courses

There are also courses that are specially designed to help you to continually develop. Information on these can be found from the Habia website and trade journals. You can also find out more by visiting the VTCT, Edexcel, and City & Guilds websites. The Connexions Direct and Directgov Careers advice websites may also be useful. You can access these websites by going to www.pearsonhotlinks.co.uk and searching for this title.

National Occupational Standards

These are the standards that describe competent performances necessary for work. The National Occupational Standards are industry-led. This means that the standards are achieved by consultations with:

- salon owners
- industry associations
- practising beauty therapists.

The National Occupational Standards are updated every few years so that they stay current. As new techniques, equipment and treatments develop and become accepted, new standards are developed.

Top tip

The National Occupational Standards help hair and beauty professionals to keep up to date with new skills and emerging trends. This in turn helps professionals to identify their future development and training needs.

Hair and Beauty Industry Authority (Habia)

Habia are the National Occupational Standards setting body for the hair and beauty industry. Visit the habia website for lots of information about the hair and beauty industry.

Memory jogger

1 What does CPD stand for?
2 What does Habia stand for?
3 What are National Occupational Standards?
4 Why is it important to manage your time at work and in your personal life?

47

Getting ready for assessment

Evidence requirements

You will be observed by your assessor on at least three occasions, two of which will cover your interaction with clients and one of which will cover your interaction with colleagues.

What you cover during your practical assessments

Ranges

From the range you must show that you have:

- participated in all the types of learning opportunity listed.

Performance criteria

In order to perform this unit successfully you must:

- develop effective working relationships with clients and colleagues
- develop yourself within your job role
- identify opportunities to learn.

What you must know

In order to pass this unit you will need to gather evidence to support a consistent performance with colleagues and clients. Assessor observation alone is not enough. You should also collect evidence to show that you have taken part in self-development activities over a period of time. This evidence will also be signed off in your candidate log book, which you will be given by your assessor. This will be an official record to show that you have covered what you need to.

Get ahead

Complete the table below by matching the qualities to the definitions.

Qualities

Committed to the beauty industry	Reliable
Conscientious	Responsible
Co-operative	Self-motivated
Dedicated	Tolerant
Flexible	Well-presented

Quality needed	Definition of the quality
	Always arriving in good time for work and not taking time off unnecessarily
	Able to adapt to different situations and circumstances without complaining
	Helpful and supportive to others; taking responsibility and making a positive contribution to the team effort
	Accepting that there is room for different views and opinions; never taking offence
	Always looking the part; projecting a professional image
	Working to high standards and being thorough
	Working safely and effectively even when unsupervised, as well as realising the importance of supervision when required
	Showing commitment to the job; being flexible and prepared to put in extra time when necessary
	Able to work well alone without needing others to organise or instruct
	Wanting to succeed as a therapist and prepared to improve standards through continuing professional development whenever the opportunity arises

UNIT B1

Prepare and maintain salon treatment work areas

Every beauty treatment and service needs a work area that is clean, tidy, hygienic and inviting. This unit is about preparing and maintaining the work area for waxing, make-up, nail, facial and eye treatments. Setting up involves preparing the tools, equipment and materials needed to carry out the treatment, as well as the seating arrangements for the client and therapist. You will also learn about the disposal of waste after treatments, client records and the importance of your personal hygiene and appearance.

In this unit you will learn how to:

- Prepare the treatment work areas
- Maintain the treatment work areas

Here are some key terms you will meet in this unit:

Disposal –
throwing away, removal

Incinerated –
disposed of by burning

Thermostatically controlled heating –
heating that is kept at a controlled temperature

Décor –
furnishings and decoration

Ventilation –
circulating fresh air

Magnifying lamp –
a lamp used in treatments that increases the size of something to make it easier to see

Disposables –
things that are meant to be thrown away after they have been used once

Flues –
outlets for fresh air

Dimmer switch –
a light switch that can be turned up or down depending on the level of lighting you want

Extractor fan –
an electric fan often set into a window and used to remove steam, fumes or stale air from a room

Equipped –
set up with the appropriate tools and equipment

Record card –
card where you write important information about the client and their treatments

Prepare the treatment work areas (1)

One of your main duties in the salon will be to assist more senior therapists by setting up the correct materials and equipment needed for a particular treatment or service and by preparing the client.

You will need to know what products, tools and equipment are needed for each of the treatments in the range, and also be able to use a client's **record card** to select materials that will be suitable for that particular client. You will also need to think very carefully about everything that you have learned about health and safety in Unit G20. Make sure your own actions reduce risks to health and safety and put it into practice.

Record cards

A client's **record card** is a professional record of treatments or services that the client has already had at your salon and is where a therapist can record comments or suggestions for future treatments. Part of your preparation for a treatment will involve obtaining a client's record card from reception. You will need the card to find out what treatment the client is booked in for, so that you know what you need to set up. The client's record card may also give you more information about the client's likes and dislikes, skin type, previous products used and the therapist's methods that will be helpful to you in deciding which products to select.

When you collect a record for a client from reception, make sure that you check the client's first name, surname and address carefully to make sure you have the correct card. Make sure that you collect the correct record for the client, as some may share a surname or even a first name.

You will need to hand over the client's record card to the therapist before she starts the treatment.

 Salon life

Jodie was looking for Mrs Jarvis's record card for the therapist, Shruti, but couldn't find it anywhere in the filing box. After five minutes she began to panic – Shruti was really strict about not starting a treatment until everything was ready, and Jodie knew that she would get into trouble if the treatment started late. Eventually the receptionist looked up from her magazine and asked Jodie what the problem was, and when Jodie explained, the receptionist told her to look under Mrs Jarvis's first name, Jan, because that's where she filed it last week. Luckily enough, there it was.

How could this problem be prevented from happening in the future?

What is the best system to use when filing record cards?

The treatment room

As the treatment room is used for a variety of different treatments, it is important that it can be adapted to meet the needs of a range of treatments and is well **equipped**.

Top tip

It is bad practice to stop a treatment in order to fetch things. This breaks the flow of the treatment and is not relaxing for the client. Whether you are setting up for a treatment you will carry out yourself or for another therapist, make sure that you have set out everything that will be needed.

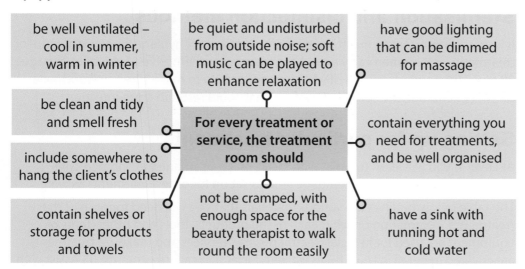

What a good treatment room should be like

You will need to bear all this in mind when preparing the treatment room.

Setting up for treatments

You need to organise the work area so that everything is hygienic and within reach and the trolley is set up with the necessary tools, equipment and products, as well as enough cotton wool and tissues. Your supervisor will show and advise you how to do this until you are able to set up on your own.

Setting up the workspace for any treatment: a checklist

1 The client's **record card** and a pen should be on the trolley ready for the consultation.

2 The gown the client will wear during the treatment should be ready, and there should be a coat hanger or hook available for the client's clothes.

3 Clean towels should be laid out nearby, either on a stool or at the end of the couch.

4 The treatment couch should be prepared with a fitted bottom sheet and a disposable couch roll.

5 The trolley tops and work surfaces should be disinfected and covered with fresh couch roll.

6 The products to be used during the treatment should be laid out on the trolley top.

7 The tools to be used during the treatment should be sterilised and then placed on the trolley top in a jar filled with antiseptic.

8 There should be enough cotton wool and tissues on the trolley to complete the whole treatment.

Get up and go!

Time yourself: set up the workspace for a treatment and record how long it takes you. In a busy salon, time is money and it is essential that assistant therapists are able to set up in time for the next client and do not hold up the appointments.

Prepare the treatment work areas (2)

Sterilisation and disinfection methods

It is just as important to maintain excellent standards of hygiene when setting up for treatments as it is when carrying out the treatments themselves. Look back at pages 20 and 21 to remind yourself of what you need to do to make sure the workspace doesn't encourage the spread of bacteria that could result in cross-infection.

Setting up for particular treatments

At Level 1, you will learn to assist with facial, make-up, manicure and pedicure treatments. However, you need to be able to set up for other treatments as well.

The table below outlines the various materials that you will need for each of these treatments. Information on what each of the products, tools and other items of equipment are used for in facial treatments, nail services and make-up treatments are covered in detail in Units B2 Assist with facial skin care treatments, B3 Assist with day make-up and N1 Assist with nail services.

Treatment	Equipment, tools and products needed
Waxing	Couch, wax station with tools, equipment and materials, protective plastic couch sheet, paper couch roll, client clothing protection, pedal waste bin, tweezers, disinfectant solution in a jar, talcum powder, cotton wool, tissues, skin-cleanser or pre-wax, medium sized towels, small scissors, selection of different sized wax strips, wax, after-wax lotion or oil, hand mirror, apron, disposable surgical gloves, pedal bin, clinical waste bin, client **record card** and pen, aftercare leaflet
Eye treatments	Couch, stool, trolley, tools, products, equipment and materials laid out, towels, tissues, orange wood sticks, head band, antiseptic cleansing solution, soothing lotion, hand mirror, damp cotton wool, dry cotton wool, scissors, tweezers, **magnifying lamp**, disposable surgical gloves, tissues, disposable spatula, steel pencil sharpener, eyebrow pencil, disinfectant solution, client **record card** and pen, pedal bin, disinfectant solution in a jar
Make-up	Couch or beauty chair, trolley, head band, tissues, couch roll, towels, hair clips, cleanser, toner and moisturiser, eye make-up remover, **magnifying lamp**, bowls, eye make-up, cheek make-up, lip make-up, foundation, powder, concealer, make-up brushes, good lighting, disposable make-up applicators, cosmetic sponges, make-up palette, pencil sharpener, spatulas, orange wood sticks, dry cotton wool, damp cotton wool, hand mirror, artificial eyelashes, client **record card** and pen
Facial	Couch, stool, trolley, facial tools, products, equipment and materials laid out, towels and **disposables** such as cotton wool, tissues, spatulas, orange wood sticks, pedal bin, disinfectant solution in a jar, head band, gown, mirror, cleansers, toners, moisturisers, massage cream or oil, exfoliants, steamer, selection of different sized bowls, comedone extractor, mask ingredients to mix or ready prepared masks, mask application brush, **magnifying lamp**, client **record card** and pen

Treatment	Equipment, tools and products needed
Manicure	Manicure station, manicure tools, bowls, finger soaking bowl, equipment and materials laid out, towels and **disposables** such as cotton wool, tissues, spatulas, emery boards and orange wood sticks, hand cream, base coat, nail polishes, top coat, cuticle knife, hoof stick, cuticle nippers, nail scissors, buffer, buffing paste, cuticle remover, cuticle massage oil or cream, hand sanitising spray, disinfectant, nail polish remover, nail polish dryer, client **record card** and pen, pedal bin, disinfectant solution in a jar
Pedicure	Pedicure station, pedicure tools, products, equipment and materials laid out, towels and **disposables** such as cotton wool, tissues, spatulas, emery boards and orange wood sticks, massage cream or foot lotion, base coat, nail polishes, top coat, cuticle knife, hoof stick, cuticle nippers, nail scissors, buffer, buffing paste, cuticle remover, cuticle massage oil or cream, hand sanitising spray, disinfectant, foot file, nail polish remover, nail polish dryer, client **record card** and pen, pedal bin, disinfectant solution in a jar
Nail art	Manicure station, medium sized towels, couch roll, dry cotton wool, tissues, hand sanitising spray, emery board, orange wood sticks, marbling tool, dotting tool, selection of nail art designs, top coat or sealant, nail polishes, nail scissors, nail polish remover, nail polish solvent, water-based and acrylic nail paints, glitter, transfers, foil strips, striping tape, jewellery, gems and rhinestones, client **record card** and pen
Nail enhancements	Nail workstation, seating, lamp, pedal bin, plastic glasses and safety mask for the nail technician, lint free pads, tissues, nail preparation products, cotton wool discs, cotton buds, orange wood sticks, cuticle knife, cuticle nippers, glass bowl, plastic bowls, dappen dish, scissors, tip cutters, coarse grit file, medium grit file, fine grit file, buffing file, four-sided buffer, medium sized towels, disinfectant solution in a jar, hand sanitising spray, nail steriliser, acetone, non-acetone polish remover, cuticle oil, client **record card** and pen

Get ahead

Find out the tools, equipment and products needed to set up for three more treatments such as massage, Indian head massage and spray tanning and write some key cards for these. Then ask a therapist if you could practise setting up for these during your work experience.

Top tip

It is helpful to have a checklist of all the tools, products and face/nail basics on a record card that you can keep nearby for reference. Cover the list with a plastic cover so that it doesn't get marked, or have it laminated so that you can wipe it clean.

Prepare the treatment work areas (3)

Environmental conditions

It is important that the environmental conditions in the treatment room are suitable for the client and the treatment. A comfortable treatment area will help to make sure that a salon visit is enjoyable for the client and a satisfying work environment for the therapist.

It is important that both the therapist and the client are comfortable

Lighting

Lighting gives a salon atmosphere, so it can have a powerful effect on how the client feels when she walks into the reception, her level of relaxation once in the treatment room, and whether she feels as though she has had a satisfying treatment at the end.

The lighting in a treatment room will depend on the treatment. For example, for make-up the lighting should be bright and not cast shadows, but for facial treatments the light should be relaxing and soft with a **magnifying lamp** available for close work and skin analysis.

The lighting should in any case be:

- bright enough to carry out treatments
- soft enough to enable clients to relax.

Therefore, it is recommended that a treatment room has a good overhead light on a **dimmer switch**, and a magnifying lamp for close work such as skin inspection.

Make sure that:

- you can always see clearly
- you and your client don't squint because lighting is poor, or become dazzled by lights that are too bright
- you always report flickering or faulty lights to your supervisor.

Heating

Clients tend to relax when they have treatments, and therefore their body temperature can drop, so it is important that the salon is warm but not so hot and stuffy that it is uncomfortable or encourages germs to multiply.

A comfortable temperature for beauty therapy work is between 20 and 24°C, with the level of moisture in the air between 40 and 60 per cent. It is also important that the salon is warm enough for clients to undress for treatments.

There are many different heating methods, but some are either too expensive to run on a regular basis or are not good at heating large areas. Therefore, the best method of heating is **thermostatically controlled heating**. This can easily be turned up or down, and every room is fitted with a radiator. When it is installed by a qualified engineer and checked annually, it is the best and most cost effective way to heat a salon.

Ventilation

Circulation of fresh air is needed to make sure that clients and staff don't become drowsy and lacking in energy as well as making sure that people are not made uncomfortable by fumes from products. Fresh air may be gained from open doors and windows, and by having an air-conditioning system in the salon.

In salons and spas that have steam and sauna areas, it is important that the air does not become too damp and humid, so good **ventilation** is essential.

If there is a lack of fresh air:

- illnesses spread because of germs and bacteria circulating around the salon
- a smelly and stuffy atmosphere is created, which is unpleasant for staff and clients
- there is a build-up of fumes from glues, varnish and cleaning products, which can cause headaches and sickness.

Methods of ventilation include **extractor fans**, windows, air vents, doors and **flues**.

General comfort

The general comfort of the client includes making sure that:

- she is seated comfortably
- she is warm
- she is happy with her surroundings
- the noise levels are not too high
- there is relaxing music playing in the background
- there are nice smells
- the **décor** is pleasant and welcoming
- the staff are polite, respectful and professional.

›› Get up and go!

Design a salon based on what you would like to see when you visit one. Think about the lighting, décor, seating and layout. Use swatches of material and colour to decorate it.

? Memory jogger

1 What is thermostatically controlled heating?

2 What can happen if there is no circulation of fresh air in the salon?

3 List five items that you would need to set up for a waxing treatment.

4 List five items that you would need to set up for a pedicure treatment.

Prepare the treatment work areas (4)

Setting up

These are the treatments that you will be involved with setting up for at Level 1.

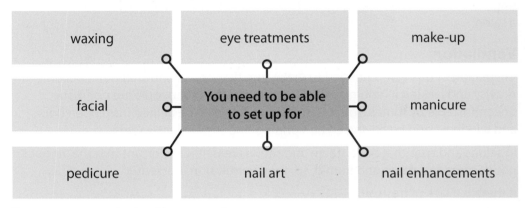

waxing	eye treatments	make-up
facial	**You need to be able to set up for**	manicure
pedicure	nail art	nail enhancements

Treatments you need to be able to set up for

As part of your assessment, you will be required to demonstrate that you are able to set up for all of these treatments.

Preparing a client for treatment

Introductions

When the client is brought through to you, or you go to collect her from reception, make sure that you have an open, confident expression. Smile and make eye contact. Greet the client by her name, then introduce yourself and explain that you will be preparing her for her treatment. Ask the client to follow you through to the treatment room. Before the treatment begins, make polite conversation to build a good relationship and help the client to feel at ease.

Polite conversation is:

- asking if she has visited the salon before
- asking if she has regular treatments
- enquiring about other treatments the client has had in the past
- enquiring whether this treatment is for a special occasion
- asking questions about the client's holidays or family
- discussing the weather or light news topics.

Polite conversation is not:

- ignoring the client in order to talk to other members of staff
- talking about yourself or another person, and not asking the client about herself
- moaning about your last client or your job
- telling the client your life story and about your problems at home
- discussing serious news topics, religion or politics.

Client care

Remove and hang up the client's coat, then show her to her seat. Make sure that she is comfortable and provide help where necessary.

Client protection

Protect the client's clothes with a towel or gown.

- For manicure: be especially careful that she is protected from varnish or other products that might stain her clothes. For protection, roll up the client's sleeves to the elbow and then tuck tissue around them.
- For make-up: protect the client's clothing with a make-up cape and protect her hair with a head band.
- For facial treatments: protect the client's upper clothing with a towel and couch roll.

Just before you start

Ask the client to remove her jewellery and show her the bowl in which you will be placing it. Point out that, if she prefers, the client (not you) could put the jewellery in her handbag.

Cleaning your hands

Explain to the client that you are going to wash your hands as this gives her confidence in your cleanliness. Make sure that you dry your hands thoroughly, because wet hands are not clean hands.

Personal presentation and behaviour

Remember that it is important to demonstrate a professional approach to all aspects of the client's visit. Your own personal presentation and behaviour are very important at all times. Looking smart and wearing appropriate protective clothing, such as a salon uniform, will give the client confidence in you. As beauty therapists are on their feet a lot and work very closely with clients, making sure that you maintain good standards of personal hygiene will mean that the client's comfort will not be affected by any body odour. You can find out more about the importance of personal presentation and behaviour on pages 24 and 25.

Appearance: a checklist

Wear smart clothes or uniform – they should be freshly laundered and not smell of smoke or strong perfume.

1 Your uniform or clothes should not be too short or too tight, and must allow for easy movement while carrying out treatments.
2 Your hair should be clean and neat.
3 Wear light, but attractive, day make-up – definitely not heavy make-up.
4 Your nails should be neatly manicured – no chipped nail varnish.
5 Keep your breath fresh – no tobacco smells.
6 If you wear jewellery, it should be simple and kept to a minimum.

? Memory jogger

1 Give two examples of polite conversation and two examples of impolite conversation.

2 Circulation of fresh air is needed to make sure that clients and staff don't become:

  A Drowsy and lacking in energy
  B Loud and talkative
  C Relaxed and chilled
  D Grumpy and irritated

3 Why should you tell your clients that you are going to wash your hands?

59

Maintain the treatment work areas (1)

It is not enough to prepare a perfect work area. It is also your responsibility to keep it clean, hygienic and looking professional at all times. To do this you must tidy up as you go along, ensure waste **disposal** is safe and, after the treatment, make sure that the area is left in a state that is suitable for the next treatment (remembering of course that it may be a different therapist and different client that could be using it next).

Safe disposal of waste

As soon as you have used cotton wool, tissues or other **disposables** you must put them in a foot pedal bin immediately. Any other type of bin is unsuitable as you will have to touch the lid to open the bin and that means your hands will not be clean and you could risk cross-infection.

For treatments such as waxing where there may be skin fluids such as blood, the waste must be disposed of in a clinical waste bin. The waste in this bin is collected by the local council and **incinerated**.

 Top tips

- Tidy up as you go – it will save time later.
- Replace bottle tops straight away.
- Place waste in the bin straight away. This is also good practice with regard to health and safety because:
  - nail varnish gives off very strong fumes
  - used cotton wool and tissues contain germs.
- During manicures and pedicures, use the nail varnish drying time to clear things away such as dirty towels and water in the manicure bowl. Clean tools and place them back in the steriliser.
- During facials, use the time when the mask is on to tidy away small items and get fresh warm water. However, you must do this very quietly so as not to disturb the client.
- If you are allowed to watch as your senior therapist is carrying out other treatments, keep an eye out for:
  - bits on the floor that may need to be put in the bin or swept up
  - tools and equipment that may need washing or disinfection
  - bottle tops that may need replacing.

Checking and cleaning equipment

The life of the equipment used depends on thorough and safe cleaning methods that follow the manufacturer's instructions. Each piece of equipment when new comes with instructions on how to clean and maintain it so that it lasts a long time. You will not be responsible for the cleaning and maintenance of equipment without supervision. However, it is your responsibility to report any possible problems that you may see with the equipment such as:

- trailing wires
- faulty plugs
- dirty machines and attachments
- broken parts.

All equipment should be checked annually by a qualified electrician. After it has been checked it will have a green safety sticker put on it which tells people that it is safe to use and has been checked. The sticker also has the date that it was tested on and when the next test is due.

Get up and go!

Find out when the equipment in your salon was last tested by a qualified electrician.

Leaving work areas clean and hygienic

When the client has left the treatment area, the following things need to be done:

- all bedding and towels washed
- products tidied away
- worktops and trolleys disinfected
- tools sterilised
- **disposables** thrown away
- equipment cleaned
- new bedding or couch roll laid out.

The exact way that things are done depends on the salon's own methods, so you will need to find out what your supervisor expects and what other things they would expect to be carried out so that the room is left in a state that is fit for the next treatment.

When you have finished the treatment, make sure that you leave the workspace perfect. It may help if you take a mental photograph of the area before you set up, which means trying to remember where and how everything was before you started and then put it back exactly how it was.

Top tip

Remember to allow a small amount of time between treatments to tidy and clean the treatment area, so that it is ready for the next client. It is bad practice for a client to enter a room or cubicle that is either unprepared or is a mess of dirty towels and has products from the last treatment spread all over the trolley.

Maintain the treatment work areas (2)

Daily and weekly cleaning

In addition to clearing and preparing the work area after a treatment, the salon furnishings and equipment should be kept clean at all times. The best way to make sure that everything is cleaned regularly is to write a list of all the cleaning jobs that need doing. There will be some jobs that need doing every day and others that are required only once a week. If a salon has an 'end-of-day' and a 'weekly' cleaning list, these jobs can be ticked off and signed each time they are done. The salon supervisor and employees can then easily check to see what cleaning jobs still need doing. The table below is an example of a daily cleaning list for a treatment room.

Daily cleaning job	Date and therapist's signature				
	23/11	24/11	25/11	26/11	27/11
Clean wax pot	SJ				
Sweep floor	SJ				
Wipe down work surfaces and trolleys	JD				
Change couch roll on trolleys	LL				
Sanitise, sterilise and put away tools	LL				
Clear away all equipment	LL				
Lay out fresh towels	JD				
Clean mirrors	SJ				

» Get up and go!

Think about the salon where you are learning or carrying out your work experience. Create a table with two columns: end-of-day cleaning and weekly cleaning. Write down as many cleaning jobs as you can think of.

When you have finished, compare your list with those of other learners in the class.

Storage of records, materials and equipment

Client records

These must be stored in line with the Data Protection Act 1998. This legislation is designed to protect client privacy and confidentiality, so all client records must be stored in a secure way such as in a lockable filing cabinet or, if stored electronically on a computer, this must be password protected.

If you are given the responsibility to put away client records, you must treat them confidentially and not show anyone the information. You must also follow the salon guidelines for storing these.

Tools and equipment

Each salon will have its own methods of safe storage of tools and equipment. However, the most important thing that you can help with is to make sure that all of these are cleaned, disinfected and sterilised before they are put away to avoid cross-contamination.

Sharp tools should always be stored so that they cannot be knocked off a shelf as they could land on someone's feet. They should also never be stored in uniform pockets.

Electrical equipment must always be turned off and unplugged when not in use and the electrical leads must not be left trailing on the floor. An important thing to remember when storing **magnifying lamps** is that they should never be left in sunlight, as this could cause a reflection that may result in a fire.

Clients' **record cards** must be stored securely

? Memory jogger

1 Under what act should client records be stored?
2 List five things that you would need to do at the end of a treatment.
3 What is the most hygienic bin to use in a salon treatment area for general treatments?
4 Why should you follow manufacturer's instructions?

 Get ahead

When an electrical appliance is checked by an electrician and a green sticker placed on it showing that it is safe to be used, what is this process called?

63

Getting ready for assessment

Evidence requirements

You will be observed by your assessor on at least three occasions and must demonstrate in your everyday work that you have met the standards for preparation and maintenance of the beauty therapy work area.

What you must cover during your practical assessments

Ranges

In your candidate log book you will have a list of ranges that you must cover during your assessment.

In this unit you must have covered the ranges below:

1 Prepared and maintained work areas for six out of the eight treatments below:

- waxing
- eye treatments
- make-up
- facial
- manicure
- pedicure
- nail art
- nail enhancements.

2 Prepared all types of environmental conditions listed below:

- lighting
- heating
- **ventilation**
- general comfort.

It is good practice to cover as many ranges as possible during each assessment. This will prevent you from having to take too many additional assessments because there are many ranges that you have not managed to cover.

Performance criteria

You must demonstrate during a practical observation by your tutor that you have:

- prepared for the treatments safely and hygienically
- considered the previous client records for further information on the set-up
- made sure that all equipment and tools have been cleaned and sterilised

- made sure that your appearance, hygiene and protection have been demonstrated
- given the correct client record to the therapist
- disposed of waste in the correct way
- checked and cleaned the equipment following the manufacturer's instructions
- cleared away and stored everything in the correct way after the treatment
- left the work area in a fit state for the next treatment.

Throughout your observations you will also need to make sure that you pay attention to health, safety and hygiene throughout, as well as presenting yourself well, so read through Unit G20 Make sure your own actions reduce risks to health and safety before any practical assessment just to refresh your memory.

Carrying out a practical treatment using unhygienic tools or without carrying out a risk assessment of your work area to avoid accidents happening will mean that you are not safe to do a treatment and therefore could mean that you do not pass your assessment or, perhaps worse, are stopped from doing your assessment.

What you must know

In order to pass this unit, you will need to gather evidence during the teaching and learning of this unit before your assessor observes your practical performance. You will gather this during class work and further study and will probably file it in a portfolio of evidence. This evidence will also be signed off in your candidate log book which you will be given by your assessor. This will be an official record to show that you have covered what you need to.

Top tips

- There is such a lot to remember when setting up for a treatment or service. Have key cards for each treatment and service that list all of the tools, products and materials required. Small record cards or postcards are a suitable size for this.
- If you are unsure about anything it is very important that you ask your supervising therapist – don't be worried about asking questions.

Salon life

Mary and Samira started work at La Belle at the same time. They were both at school most of the week and spent one day a week at the salon. It was a very busy salon and there was always so much to do to help the senior therapists. Mary loved the work but felt that she ended up doing most of the clearing up and Samira got the better job of preparing the rooms. Not only that, because Samira did the setting-up the senior therapists praised her all the time because they loved the organised, fresh-smelling rooms that they took their clients into. Unfortunately they didn't notice Mary: by the time she had cleaned out the rooms, collected the laundry and emptied the bins it was time for Samira to do her bit, lighting candles, preparing cotton wool and tissues and changing the music. It all just seemed a little unfair, but Mary didn't want to make a fuss. Mary had asked Samira if they could share the different jobs, but Samira had a way with words and said that Mary had the most important role.

Do you think that this would be a fair share of duties in the salon? If not, why?

How would you deal with this situation if it happened to you?

UNIT G2

Assist with salon reception duties

Although some salons employ an experienced receptionist who is not a beauty therapist, it is more usual for existing beauty staff to take turns in running reception. Assisting with salon reception duties will involve keeping the reception clean, tidy and organised, making appointments, attending to clients, selling products and handling money. You will be able to use your knowledge of treatments and products to give clients good advice, and assisting with reception will also help you to improve your understanding of the working pressures that therapists experience.

Many clients will decide whether or not they like a salon within moments of arriving in the reception area, so you need to make sure that the client's first and lasting impression is a good one. Communication skills are very important, and you need to be enthusiastic, cheerful, helpful, professional and respectful to every client. By doing a good job with assisting with reception, you will contribute to the successful running and good reputation of your salon.

In this unit you will learn how to:

- Maintain the reception area
- Attend to clients and enquiries
- Help to make appointments for salon services

66

Here are some key terms you will meet in this unit:

Professional – high standards and a good attitude

Respectful – treating others with politeness and thought

Discreet – careful in your choice of words, loudness of speech and able to act in a confidential manner

Confidential – keeping things private

Slang – informal language and speech

Potential clients – people who are interested in beauty treatments and may use the salon in the future

Authority – the limits of your power and what you are allowed to do

Confidentiality – keeping all personal information that a client tells you private

Stock rotation – bringing the older stock items to the front of the display or for use and placing the new ones at the back

Shelf life – the life of the product before it passes its sell-by date

Formal – speaking or acting respectfully in a way that is not familiar to someone

Complementary therapies – treatments such as reflexology aromatherapy and Indian head massage that were originally from different cultures or countries

Maintain the reception area (1)

Remember that the reception area is the first point of contact for clients. Although the booking of appointments, both on the telephone and in person, is obviously a key purpose of a reception area, there are many other reasons why a beauty salon needs a reception.

- It is where information and help on treatments and products are provided.
- It is where the sale of products and the handling of money for product sales and treatments take place.
- It is used for handing out brochures and price lists to **potential clients**.
- Window and cabinet display for products, and possibly even flower displays, will be set up here.
- It is where clients are looked after, both before and after treatment.

Maintaining the reception area will involve attention to all these things.

The reception area from outside

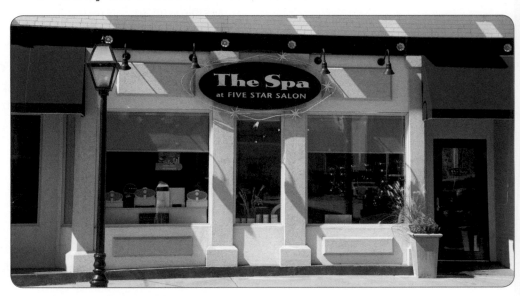

The outside of the beauty salon should encourage people to want to enter

For people in the street – who may be potential clients – the reception area is an extension of the shop window. As they look into the salon, they will see the reception area. It is therefore important that this area appears organised and very clean, and gives a good impression of the salon.

The shop front should encourage clients to enter, so ideally it will have:

- plants or hanging baskets
- information about the salon's hours of opening
- signs saying what treatments are available
- clean windows
- a freshly painted exterior – not cracked or peeling
- a well-swept front.

Get ahead

Design your own reception area. Think about what you need and where everything should be placed. Design it by creating a virtual reception either on the computer or by making a model using swatches of material and colour schemes.

However, although it is good to have a central position in a busy shopping area for a beauty salon, it is best not to be in full view of passing people. Blinds can therefore be used to screen waiting clients from public view and to shade display products from the hot sun.

Inside the reception area

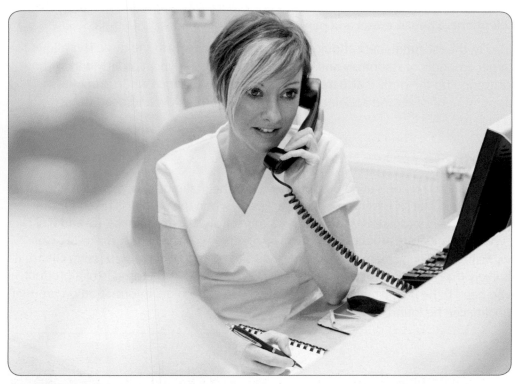

The salon reception desk should be neat and tidy at all times

When a client enters the reception area, he or she needs to feel welcome and at ease with the staff and surroundings. It is also important that clients have the impression that the salon is being run **professionally** and efficiently.

The whole reception area should be well lit, warm, fresh-smelling and, most importantly, spotless. There should be a comfortable seating area for waiting clients with a selection of up-to-date magazines and promotion leaflets. The temperature should be warm in the cooler seasons and airy in the summer months. Refreshments in the form of tea, coffee and mineral water should be available for clients, both before and after treatment. Soothing background music should be played to create a relaxed atmosphere and enhance clients' experience of the salon.

In the reception area there should be a locked product display cabinet from which clients can view and purchase skin, body and nail care products. All salon staff should be familiar with the products so that they can advise clients. If you notice that stocks are low, inform the correct staff member.

The décor of the salon should reflect the image that the salon wants to achieve. The colours and textures of the walls, ceilings, furniture, linen and towels should work together to create the correct atmosphere of tranquility and relaxation. A more modern and funky approach to design is not recommended as it can date very quickly. It is best to aim for a classic design, using pale colours for a fresh look.

>> **Get up and go!**

What beauty salons are there in your area? Have you visited them? If you have, think about their reception area, what they do right and what they could improve on. Discuss in pairs or as a group.

Maintain the reception area (2)

Stationery and paperwork

The reception desk should be positioned so that the receptionist can greet everyone that enters the salon. It should be neat and tidy at all times with just the essentials on view – the cash till, the appointment book, price lists, appointment cards, the telephone, a pencil, eraser and pen.

Ideally, the reception desk should have shelving underneath the desk. This allows for larger amounts of stationery and paperwork to be stored in an orderly way without cluttering up the desk. It also makes it easy to see at a glance when brochures, appointment cards and appointment sheets are getting low and need to be reordered.

Products

Beauty salons rely on selling products to boost their takings and, although all staff are involved, the sale is completed at reception when the money is taken for the product. The typical items that beauty salons sell are skin care, make-up and nail care products. These are attractive products to clients – we all love new make-up, nail varnishes and skin creams. If attractively displayed and on show to passing clients, it is likely that these products will sell easily. In order to assist in the sale of a product, you need to be familiar with the prices offered in your salon. Information on product pricing can be found on page 77.

> **Top tip** ✓
>
> If you notice that salon stationery is getting low, take responsibility and inform the member of staff who deals with stock and ordering.

A product display

Product display

The best way to display products is in the reception area in a locked glass-fronted cabinet. The cabinet should be positioned away from the glare and direct heat of the sun. This is because the heat could:

- bleach the boxes
- cause the products to thicken and separate.

The products should be neatly arranged and clearly visible to the eye. There should be enough items on display to catch people's interest without them looking cluttered. One or two of each item that you stock is enough.

The products should look as new as when they were first put on display. It is therefore important that they are taken out and dusted regularly. If the products are dusty or look old, it will discourage people from buying them. Keep an eye out for any damage, loose packaging, cracks and leaks – you will need to remove any breakages or faulty products from the display cabinet and report them straight away to the relevant person.

The stock cupboard

The main stock should be stored out of view, but in an easy-to-reach location, so that when a sale is made the product can be accessed easily. It is also good for the client to see that she is purchasing a new product and not one that has been used for display purposes.

Correct storage of stock

To prevent spoilage and extend a product's **shelf life**, it should generally be kept:

- dry and cool
- in a dark place away from sunlight
- away from naked flames
- in an airtight container – for example, if you open a face cream and then try to reseal it, it will be unfit for sale.

However, you should always check the manufacturer's instructions about correct product storage.

Product shelf life

Remember that all stock has a shelf life. This means that it has a recommended time limit during which it should be stored or used. After this time, the product can go off, making it unfit for use and unsellable to customers. Outward signs that a product has gone off are:

- an unpleasant smell
- separation – this is when a cream or lotion is no longer completely mixed together and becomes part cream, part liquid
- thickness – if a product has passed its sell-by date or has been open to the air, it can turn hard where it becomes dehydrated
- discolouration – this is when a product changes colour.

Maintain the reception area (3)

Products

Stock rotation

To make sure that products are used within their **shelf life** and do not go off, a system known as **stock rotation** is used.

- New stock received from suppliers is placed at the back of the storage area so that it is sold last.
- Stock already on the premises is stored at the front and is sold first.

If your salon does not sell a lot of stock, then products will be sitting in storage for some time and sell-by dates will need to be checked on a regular basis and less stock carried. When stock is reaching its sell-by date, salons usually promote it as a special offer and sell it at a discounted price.

> **» Get up and go!**
>
> Think of a beauty product that you would like to sell. To make sure stock is sold before its sell-by date, you are going to advertise this product at a discounted price and design a 'special offer' poster to be displayed in the reception area. The special offer could be a percentage or a half-price discount, or a buy-one-get-one-free offer.
>
> Remember to make the poster colourful, tasteful and easy to read. It must be eye-catching.

Recording stock levels

Stock should be checked in and out of the salon using either a stock sheet (the manual method) or a computer (a computerised system). If stock levels are not recorded properly, it is impossible to know when to reorder products and which ones to reorder. It is also impossible to check which products are popular with clients and whether any have been stolen.

When stock is counted on a regular basis, this is called a stock take.

Stock taking

When carrying out a stock take, there should be a list of available stock for sale and salon use, either in a file, a stock sheet or on the computer. All staff should record when a new product is opened for use in the salon, and when an old product is empty and the bottle or tub is discarded. They should also keep a record of any sales and breakages. Ideally, a stock take should be done each week so that available stock is counted and a list made of new stock to be ordered. A stock take is best done using a stock sheet.

Using a stock sheet

When new stock arrives in the salon, each individual item needs to be entered into the amount column. It is not advisable to enter the total amount of stock in one cell, as this would make it difficult to count out. For example, if you receive four cleansers, you should mark '1' in the amount column four times. In this way, stock can easily be checked out by crossing through each '1'.

Once you have entered the product and the amount of stock, then you can complete the column for 'Date in'. When stock is removed from the stock cupboard, you should complete the columns for 'Date out' and 'Reason'.

Product	Date in	Amount	Date out	Reason	Signature
Cleanser for dry skin	20/09/10	I I I	28/09/10	sale	SJT
		I I I I I			
		I I			
		I			
Toner for dry skin	20/09/10	I	01/10/10	damaged – reported	LL
		I			

An example of a simple stock sheet

Possible reasons for stock out that you may put on the stock sheet are:

- sale
- display
- salon use
- damaged or broken.

The person who has removed the stock must sign in the 'Signature' column. When more stock that is new arrives, enter it in the space at the bottom of the chart with the date, so it is obvious which entries are new and which are old stock.

» Get up and go!

You have noticed the following problems:

- a damaged product
- low stationery
- there is only one moisturiser for sensitive skin remaining in the cabinet.

Who do you report these problems to?

Using information from your place of work or your training school or college, write out and complete the table below. You may want to add any other things that need reporting.

Problem to report	Member of staff to report to
Low on price lists and appointment cards	
Broken products	
Damaged goods	
Low on make-up and skin care products	

? Memory jogger

1 What is stock rotation?

2 What is shelf life?

3 What is a stock take?

4 What is a product display?

Attend to clients and enquiries (1)

When you are assisting on reception, you are the first point of contact for every person who enters your salon. You are on show to everyone, and so your appearance, attitude and communication skills are very important. Remember that working in the beauty industry involves helping clients to feel relaxed and better about themselves, and so you need to be polite, positive and attentive at all times when attending to the visitors to your salon and listening to their enquiries.

Personal presentation

It is essential that your appearance is of a very high standard. Most clients will think that the way the receptionist appears reflects the standards in the salon. If the staff are sloppy and untidy in appearance, then a client may think that the salon is sloppy and untidy too. Some tips on how to ensure that your appearance is **professional** can be found in Units G20 and G3.

Communication

As a receptionist, you will be greeting clients; booking appointments; answering queries; selling products; dealing with complaints; answering the telephone; taking messages and passing on information, perhaps from a client to a therapist, or from a therapist to a client, or from one member of your team to another. Being able to communicate positively and effectively is essential to your role.

There are different forms of communication:

- Oral – speaking to another person. This includes speaking by telephone or face-to-face conversations.
- Body language – eye contact, nodding or smiling, for example; not spoken language.
- Visual – pictures that communicate information such as adverts, posters, magazines and brochures.
- Written – for example, letters, memos, faxes, text messages and email.

Communicating effectively involves making use of all of these methods and knowing which method to use for a particular situation. Often you will use a combination of methods. Your body language and the way you say things can be just as important as the words you use. In Unit G3 Contribute to the development of effective working relationships you learned about positive and negative communication. Think about some of the examples of negative communication, such as yawning or slouching. If you were feeling tired or worried about a personal issue, you might communicate a negative message to a client without meaning to. You must always maintain a **professional** attitude.

You must also remember that effective communication is a two-way process. It is about receiving as well as giving information. Its success depends on how clearly we can make ourselves understood as well as how clearly we can understand others. Noting down information, being prompt when passing on messages and using clear language when you speak are all very important, but so too are listening carefully to what other people say and interpreting any other messages that someone might be trying to communicate to you. Do all that you can to make sure that you communicate as clearly as possible.

Top tip

It is very rude and unprofessional to keep a client waiting without keeping her fully informed of what is going on. If a client realises that she will not be dealt with immediately, then she can decide whether to wait in the salon or return later. If a client is not kept informed of this, she may become impatient and unhappy.

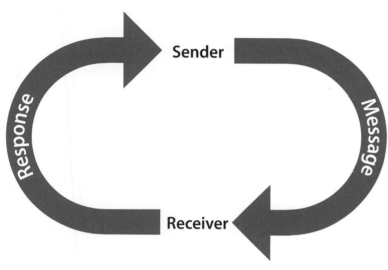

The process of communication

Get up and go!

Below is a list of some of the different tasks that a receptionist may need to communicate. Think about each task and identify the best method of communication to use for each of them. Some of the methods are quicker than others, so you will need to prioritise. In other words, decide how important or urgent the message is, then decide on the best method of communication.

You may like to copy the table below then draw a line to connect each task with the correct method as they are not in the correct order.

Task	Method of communication
To let a therapist know that her next client has cancelled an appointment	Invoice
To inform all staff of the extended opening times in the salon	Meeting
To let all staff know about the reception duty rota	Memo
To tell customers about new products	Notice board
To inform a client how much she owes	Leaflet
To bill a customer for her course of treatments	Spoken word

75

Attend to clients and enquiries (2)

Welcoming clients

The value of a warm welcome for clients must not be underestimated – a cheerful and bright smile that is genuine will instantly put a client at ease, whether she has arrived for an appointment or to make an enquiry.

- A **professional** yet welcoming greeting would be: 'Good morning/afternoon Ms/Mrs/Miss/Mr ...' (use the client's name if you know it). 'How can I be of help?'
- A professional goodbye would be: 'We hope to see you again soon. Goodbye Ms/Mrs/Miss/Mr ...' (while holding the door open for the person).

Welcoming clients: a checklist

1 Make eye contact without staring and keep your facial expressions open – don't frown, roll your eyes or glare.

2 Don't chat to other members of staff while a client is with you, unless it is to answer an enquiry about their appointment or treatment.

3 Vary the tone of your voice so that you don't sound bored and disinterested. Ask helpful questions to show interest in your client.

4 Be caring and **discreet**. Remember, many clients feel quite nervous about visiting a beauty salon.

Taking the client's money

A very important part of being on a reception desk is taking the client's payment for treatment. There are many different methods and it takes a while to be able to carry out the different ways accurately and efficiently, especially if the reception is very busy. You will not be expected to do this alone. A senior colleague or receptionist will instruct and help you to make sure that you can do it properly as it is an extremely responsible job and very easy to make mistakes.

Types of payment

Products or treatment can be paid for with cash, cheques, credit cards, debit cards or gift vouchers.

When taking money it is always a good idea to say to the client how much the product or treatment is, state how much money they give you, and then give the receipt and/or change to the client, stating this amount also.

Confirming appointments

A client who has arrived for an appointment is referred to as an 'existing booking'. When a client arrives for an appointment, take the client's appointment details, confirm them with her and have them checked by a senior staff member. Ask the client to take a seat in the reception area, and offer her magazines and refreshments

Top tip

Concentrate on your numeracy and ICT skills. Numeracy skills are very important for work on a reception. Taking payment, pricing products and working out time needed for appointments all need you to use maths. ICT skills are also important as many tills and client record systems are electronic.

in line with your salon's policy. Then inform the therapist who will be treating her that her next client has arrived.

Client enquiries

To be in a good position to deal with client enquiries, you need to know about the treatments offered in your salon, how long each treatment takes, which therapists can offer them, how much they cost and the benefits they offer, as well as information about the different products that are available for clients to buy. Your supervisor or manager will guide you as you learn how to deal with these sorts of enquiries.

The most common types of treatments and services offered are:

- manicures
- pedicures
- waxing
- facials
- eye treatments such as brow shaping, lash and brow tinting
- body massage
- ear piercing
- nail extensions
- spray tanning.

Some salons also offer **complementary therapies** such as:

- aromatherapy
- reflexology
- hot stone therapy
- Indian head massage.

Service pricing

Prices of treatments and services vary a great deal across different towns, cities and regions of the UK, so it is important to become familiar with the prices of the treatments offered in the salon that you work in.

Product pricing

As with services, product pricing varies, so again it is important that you are familiar with the prices of the products offered in your salon. Prices are usually set by working out:

- cost price – the price the salon buys the product at
- an additional mark-up that the salon decides in order to make a profit
- these two things will result in a recommended retail price (RRP).

For example:

Nail varnish: Cost price £5.50 + salon mark-up £4.00 = RRP £9.00

» Get up and go!

Calculate the following:

- A client's bill comes to £58 and she wants to book and pay for a pedicure for her friend next week which costs £30.
- She wants to pay for her bill using two different methods of payment: a gift voucher for £25 plus the rest on her credit card.
- How much would she need to pay on her credit card?

77

Attend to clients and enquiries (3)

Giving information on products and services

Below are some examples of questions that a client might ask about beauty treatments and products.

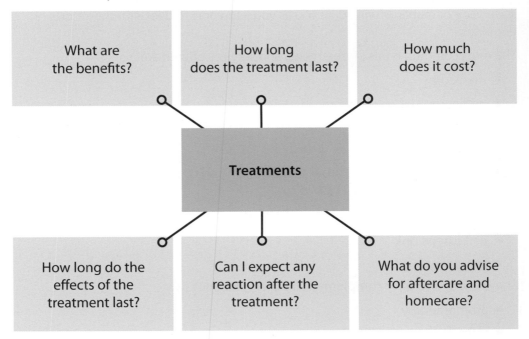

Questions clients might ask about a treatment

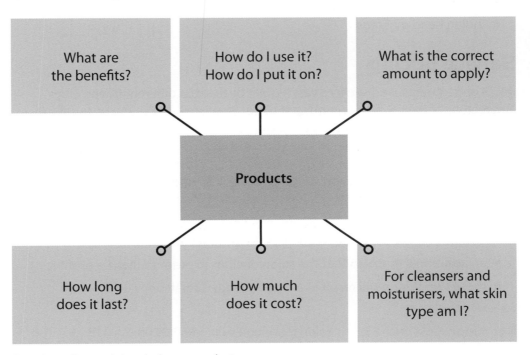

Questions clients might ask about a product

Products for sale

 Get up and go!

In pairs, choose a product and learn about it for 10–15 minutes.

Now test your knowledge. One of you will be the client, the other will be the therapist. The client asks the therapist questions about the product, for the therapist to answer. When you have finished, swap roles and repeat this activity for a treatment.

How much did you know? Imagine having to give information about all the products and treatments that are available in a beauty salon.

It takes time and practice to be able to advise clients on the different products for sale and the type of treatments available. As a trainee, you can expect to be asked many questions to which you will not know the answer but, with time, the help of your manager and perseverance on your part, you will gradually learn what the best advice to give is.

You may also receive enquiries from suppliers, but you will not have the **authority** to deal with these apart from taking a message to pass on to the appropriate person. It is important to act **professionally** and use good communication techniques when dealing with all visitors and enquiries to the salon.

When dealing with enquiries and requests, it is essential that you keep within the limits of your own authority. There will be many times when you need to pass an enquiry or request on to a senior member of staff. For example, if one of the salon's suppliers needs to speak to the manager but she is at lunch and won't return for ten minutes, you should offer the supplier a coffee, show him or her the list of products that the manager wrote down in the morning, and explain that the manager will confirm what is needed when she returns from lunch.

✓ **Top tip**

It is best to refer a client to a senior member of staff rather than give out incorrect information. The consequences of giving a client incorrect information could be a reaction to a product, a returned product, or a client complaint.

 Memory jogger

1 What enquiries might you have on reception?
2 What other skills might be useful while working on reception?
3 List three general beauty treatments that might be booked on reception.
4 List three complementary beauty treatments that might be booked on reception.

Attend to clients and enquiries (4)

Dealing with complaints

When a complaint is made, the reception desk is normally the first point of contact. From there, the complaint will be passed on to the appropriate senior member of staff. As there will probably be clients waiting in reception while someone makes a complaint, it is very important that complaints are dealt with politely and without aggression. It would be embarrassing for waiting clients, and give a very poor impression of the salon, if a complaint was not handled well.

Most people dread having to deal with a complaint. Some people are very good at calming down an angry client or tackling a difficult situation. Other people react in a way that only seems to make the situation worse.

You will not be expected to sort out a complaint until much further into your training. While you are a trainee, you should pass the complaint on to the correct member of staff.

Most complaints can be sorted out quickly and easily because most clients are reasonable and know exactly what will make them happy again. On rare occasions, however, you may experience a more difficult situation that tests your patience. Whatever the situation, the client making the complaint should be gently moved away from the reception area into a quieter area of the salon, where the complaint can be dealt with privately.

Top tips ✓

- Watch and learn from your workmates. You will see good and bad ways of dealing with a complaint.
- A client who complains is giving you a second chance. An unhappy client who doesn't complain will probably tell others how dissatisfied she is and never return.

Having a positive influence

When dealing with complaints, there are qualities and skills that will help to solve the problem in the best way. These are:

- patience
- acting on a complaint, not reacting
- listening skills
- deciding on the main facts
- remaining calm
- keeping an open expression
- positive body language.

You can have a positive influence

Don't forget that one of the most important and effective ways to deal with a complaint is to apologise to the client for the fact that she is unhappy with the situation. Your client could be unhappy with:

- how he or she has been treated
- the standard of treatment
- an incorrect appointment
- a faulty product that he or she purchased
- an unpleasant skin reaction to a treatment or product.

An apology will go a long way to helping your client feel better about the situation and the treatment received from the salon.

Answering the telephone

When assisting on reception, you will have to answer the telephone. Remember that answering the telephone at work is not the same as speaking on the phone to friends or family. Take care to pronounce words clearly, using good communication skills, and never use **slang**. Smile! Even though the other person can't see you, you will sound friendlier.

The most acceptable method of telephone greeting is to use a polite greeting first, add the name of the salon, and then ask how you can help. Each salon usually has a preferred method of greeting when answering the telephone, and they will train their staff in this. It is good to be polite and **respectful** without being too **formal**.

Taking messages

You will frequently be asked to take messages during your time on reception. This must be done promptly, accurately and in writing that is neat and easy to read.

Details that you will need to write are:

- the date and time of the message or call
- who the message is from
- who the message is for
- what the message is about
- how important the message is – urgent, important or no immediate hurry
- the caller's name, company name and contact details (telephone number).

It is very important that you remember to write down all this information, because any details that are missed could result in a complete misunderstanding. Don't rely on memory. When the salon is busy and you have lots of other things to remember, it is easy to forget the details of a message.

Top tip

Message pads can help to jog a person's memory. These list all the information you should write down when taking a message and can be purchased from stationery shops.

Get up and go!

Design your own message sheet. You may like to do this by hand or on a computer. When you have finished, photocopy the sheet a few times. You may like to use it when you are on reception to see how it works.

Attend to clients and enquiries (5)

Confidentiality

Remember that, as a receptionist, you are in a position of responsibility and there are certain salon and legal requirements that you must meet.

Confidentiality is central to the running of a **professional** beauty salon. A client must feel confident that any personal information she gives remains private and that the staff don't gossip about her behind her back. Gossiping about clients is unprofessional behaviour that breaks a client's trust and is extremely disrespectful to the client.

What information is confidential?

Confidential information

 Top tip

Information is given by a client to a therapist or receptionist in confidence. This information must remain private unless it is illegal or could hurt someone. If you are unsure or worried about confidentiality, always check with your manager.

Record systems

Confidential information, such as client records, should never be visible to other clients or to members of staff not treating the client. They should be stored in lockable drawers underneath the reception desk.

While on reception duty, you will see clients' private records. You have no right to pass these on or to talk about them to anyone, except other members of staff who need to know because they may carry out a treatment on or look after the client. Even then, you must only discuss client details when it concerns a work-related matter and you have the permission of the client. If you are unsure about what to do, ask a senior member of staff.

The Data Protection Act 1998

The Data Protection Act covers many different working practices. The section that is important to beauty therapists is the one that describes the correct privacy methods that should be in place in a salon. These privacy methods ensure that it is difficult for other people to get hold of, look at or use a person's private details without permission, for any reason.

The act states that beauty therapists should treat a client's personal details in confidence – that means keeping it private. It is against the law to give out someone's personal information without his or her permission.

Top tips

- Never leave a record card on the reception desk in full view of everyone.
- Never allow clients to view a person's record card on a computer screen.

Get up and go!

Use the Internet to find out more about the Data Protection Act 1998 and how it affects the beauty industry.

Salon life

It was a very busy Saturday morning in the salon. The reception was buzzing with clients waiting for treatments and buying products. Li-ying noticed a woman hovering outside the door looking very unsure of herself. She wondered whether the woman wanted to see a brochure or book a treatment, or whether she was just waiting for someone. Li-ying wasn't sure what she should say to her.

Then Lisa, the salon junior, called to the woman over the heads of the other clients, saying 'Come in, we don't bite!' The woman came in rather sheepishly. Li-ying asked, 'How can we help?' The woman explained in a whispered voice that she was interested in waxing. 'What part of the body?' called out Lisa from the other end of the desk. The woman winced. She didn't want to say in front of all the other people, so took a brochure and hurried out saying that she would telephone later.

Could this matter have been dealt with better? If so, how?

Was the communication between the potential client and the staff good? Why?

Do you think that the woman will return to the salon? Give a reason for your answer.

? Memory jogger

1 What is confidential information?

2 Why must you store record cards or other confidential information in line with the Data Protection Act?

3 List three qualities and skills that are needed when dealing with complaints.

Help to make appointments for salon services [1]

One of your key tasks when assisting on reception will be to help make appointments. Booking appointments is not an easy thing to do. Mistakes can happen very easily, and very small mistakes in the appointment columns can cause huge problems for the salon staff, such as double bookings, lack of time to finish a treatment and clients left waiting. This can then in result in a stressful environment where there are unhappy clients, overworked therapists and embarrassed staff.

Booking basics

Salon appointments are recorded on loose sheets of paper, in an appointment book, or on an electronic record system on a computer. Paper appointment sheets contain several columns. At the top of each column, the name of the therapist is entered. The receptionist and other staff can then see clearly at a glance:

- which therapist is treating which client at which time
- which therapist has room for more appointments
- who is taking breaks and when.

The appointment pages are created or written up weeks in advance because appointments can be made months ahead, for example if a client is having a course of treatments. Another reason may be that a client wishes to book for a special occasion such as a pre-wedding pamper, and will therefore need to book a certain date and time months in advance. Writing up the weeks ahead also helps staff to plan their holidays and work timetables can then be organised around them.

Date: Tuesday 13th October 2009

	Lucy	Hellena	Anetta	Siobhan	
AM 9.00	Mrs Khan	Mrs Hughes			9.00 AM
9.15	full	full			9.15
9.30	Body wax	B/Massage			9.30
9.45	01234 45678	223335			9.45
10.00					10.00
10.15					10.15
10.30		Mrs Inder			10.30
10.45	Miss Jones	Pedicure			10.45
11.00	Aroma	+ 1/2 leg wax	Miss Westerby		11.00
11.15	Back massage	01235 771540	French		11.15
11.30	357928		Manicure		11.30
11.45			+ facial		11.45
12.00			01329 815242	Mr. Vallete	12.00
12.15		Mrs Green		Back massage	12.15
12.30	LUNCH	Eye tint		+ pedicure	12.30
12.45		444321		02271 881570	12.45
PM 1.00	Mr. Walsh				1.00 PM
1.15	Manicure		Miss Rudman		1.15
1.30	+back wax	LUNCH	Miss Allen	Miss Binder	1.30
1.45	02392 815815		x2 eyebows	waxing	1.45
2.00	Mrs Suling		335215	e/b + lip & chin	2.00
2.15	Eyebrow tidy	Miss Murphy	LUNCH	07807 577211	2.15
2.30	413927	Arm wax			2.30
2.45		+ u/arm wax			2.45
3.00		223792	Miss Nair	Mrs Pattel	3.00
3.15			Bridal	Sugaring	3.15
3.30		Miss Woolford	Top to toe	to x2 leg	3.30
3.45		Basic facial +	447 812	221 335	3.45
4.00	Mrs Wang	eye lash tint			4.00
4.15	Non-surg.	445 877			4.15
4.30	facial lift				4.30
4.45	08789 815 111				4.45
5.00		Mrs Townsend			5.00
5.15		M/up			5.15
5.30		lesson			5.30
5.45		315579 ext. 222			5.45
6.00					6.00
6.15					6.15
6.30					6.30
6.45					6.45
7.00					7.00

lunchtime cover only

A page from an appointment book

Making a booking

A client may make a booking over the telephone, in person at the salon, by text or online. Electronic methods of booking are becoming much more popular.

The first thing you need to do is to take the client's details. You will need to find out the following.

- The client's surname and first initial. It is not advisable to write first names because other members of staff may not know the client by their first name, nor is it a good idea to just put a surname because there may be other clients with that name. If you write the client's first initial and surname, it is easy for a therapist to look up that person's details on a record card should they need to contact the client about the booking. Another reason for using the client's surname is that some clients do not like being called by their first name.
- The client's telephone number. Make sure that you write the dialing code if the telephone number is not a local one. You should also take down the client's work number if this is where the client can be contacted during working hours.
- The client's treatment. This is usually written in using an abbreviation.

Imagine if a first name only was entered into the appointment book, and the incorrect telephone number was written down. How could you try to contact the client to cancel her appointment if, for example, the therapist was ill?

If your salon uses an appointment book, follow this advice when writing in the columns.

- Appointments must be written in pencil only so that mistakes or changes can be rubbed out. Don't press too hard with the pencil as it makes it hard to rub out.
- Your writing should be neat, clear and small. This is to allow room for all the client and treatment details to be written in a small space.
- It is better to print words, rather than write in a joined up style, especially if your handwriting is not very good.

 Top tip

If you are ever uncertain while helping on reception, ask for help. This is not a sign of failure; it shows that you are acting sensibly, and will help you to avoid making a double booking or an incorrect booking which then leads to an incorrect treatment.

» Get up and go!

Design a client questionnaire to gain feedback from clients on how they think you performed while on reception duty. Make the questionnaire quite simple and short as clients may not have much time to complete it.

Identifying the client's requirements

When a client contacts you to make an appointment, let her tell you exactly what she would like before interrupting her. If the client only has an idea, then help her to decide. Then repeat the information to check that you have correctly understood her wishes. If you have the **authority** to book the treatment, then you can do so.

Help to make appointments for salon services (2)

Making a new booking

Here are the steps to booking an appointment in person or by telephone under the guidance of a senior staff member:

1 Ask what treatment the client would like to book and when.

2 Ask if the client would like to see a particular therapist.

3 Look at the appointment book and offer some available dates and times.

4 When the day, date and time have been agreed, write the client's name, telephone number and treatment in pencil only.

5 Read back the day, date, time and therapist to the client to make sure that no mistakes have been made. This part is very important.

6 Write down the appointment details on an appointment card to give to the client.

7 Get the senior member of staff to check the entry before the client leaves.

New booking procedure

Top tip

When making an appointment, make sure that you write in the column as you confirm the day, date and time to a client. Never write this information in the column after putting down the telephone or after the client has left the salon – this is asking for trouble. Another client could come in, the phone could ring again, a senior therapist could ask you to do some jobs for her, by which time you will have forgotten all about the appointment that you should have written down.

What to do when problems arise:

- If the time that the client wants is not free, then offer the nearest time to it.

- If the client wants to see a certain therapist, but that therapist is already booked, then offer the client the next and nearest time available for that therapist. If that time is not convenient, then offer the client a different therapist.

- If an appointment needs to be changed, rub it out and rewrite it in the book and on the client's appointment card.

Booking out time for treatments

Another factor to think about is how long to book out for each treatment. Your manager will need to tell you how this is done for your salon, and show you how to do it. However, on nearly every appointment sheet, one line in a column stands for a 15-minute time slot. For example, if a facial takes one hour to complete, then four lines will need to be crossed through in a column.

When booking out some appointments, time should be allowed for client preparation, consultation, homecare and aftercare advice. You should therefore book out treatment time and add 15 minutes (one line) if needed. Examples are given in the table on page 89.

As a beauty therapist becomes more experienced at giving treatments, she will probably work more quickly and will not need all the time put aside for a treatment. She would therefore have enough time for preparation, consultation and advice, without the need for the receptionist to book out extra time for this. Extra time for preparation, consultation and advice is needed mainly for larger, more relaxing treatments such as facials, body massages and complementary therapies.

Help to make appointments for salon services (3)

Commercially acceptable treatment times

There are set times for treatments known as commercially acceptable treatment times. This is how long a treatment should take in order to make a salon money.

It is important to bear in mind these times when you are taking bookings. Some therapists work slightly slower or quicker than others, but still manage to complete their treatments within an acceptable time. Each therapist should let the receptionist know exactly how long she needs for each treatment.

More information on commercially acceptable treatment times can be found under Treatment times and prices on pages 214–215.

Treatment codes

As there is not much space for writing appointment details in the columns, abbreviated codes are used to show which treatment has been booked. These codes vary from salon to salon, but are usually quite similar. Treatment codes are shown in the last column of the table on page 89.

When not to book an appointment

It is rewarding to have responsibility, but remember that there is a limit to your **authority**. It is important that you do not carry out activities without the permission and guidance of a senior staff member. Appointment systems can be tricky to master and easy to mess up, so ask for help where necessary. Always check appointments with a senior staff member until you have been given permission to carry out bookings on your own.

However, there will be certain treatments or clients that you will never be allowed to book. Examples of these are given in the table below. Always pass these cases on to a senior member of staff.

When not to book a client	Reason why
A course of treatments	This needs careful thought and planning by the therapist carrying out the course of treatments, so the booking is best done by the therapist.
An electrical treatment such as electrolysis	More thorough consultation and advice are needed before a client is allowed to have electrical treatments. Sometimes a doctor's permission is needed.
A person under the age of 16 without a parent present	This is for insurance reasons and to check that the client has parental permission.
If a client cannot give you a contact telephone number	You would be unable to contact the client if there was a problem with the booking and you needed to change or cancel it, for example due to staff illness.
If a client comes in who has been disruptive and rude on a previous visit	A disruptive client will upset both staff and other clients.

Top tips ✓

If a client wishes to make an appointment when a senior staff member is busy, you will not have the authority to do this. Explain that you need help as you are learning. If you feel confident enough to make the booking, explain that you must get it checked afterwards.

›› Get up and go!

Copy and complete the table below to show lines to cross through treatment codes. Complete this information for pedicures through to ear piercing.

Treatment	Maximum time allowed in minutes without consultation time	Preparation/consultation time	Number of lines to cross through in appointment sheet/book	Treatment code
Eyebrow shape	15 minutes	0 – advise while treating	1	EBS
Eyelash tint	20 minutes	0 – advise while treating	2	ELT
Facial	45 minutes	1 – for undressing, aftercare advice and tidying of work area	4	FAC
Make-up	45 minutes	0 – advise while treating	3	M-UP
Manicure	30 minutes	0 – advise while treating	2	MAN
Pedicure	45 minutes	1 – to allow drying time and putting on of shoes, also tidying of work area		
Eyebrow wax	15 minutes	0 – advise while treating		
Underarm wax	15 minutes	0 – advise while treating		
Half leg wax	30 minutes	0 – advise while treating		
Bikini wax	15 minutes	0 – advise while treating		
Arm wax	30 minutes	0 – advise while treating		
Full leg wax	50 minutes	0 – advise while treating		
Half leg, bikini and underarm wax	60 minutes	0 – advise while treating		
Full leg, bikini and underarm wax	75 minutes	0 – advise while treating		
Eyebrow shape and eyelash tint	35 minutes	0 – advise while treating		
Eyebrow tint	10 minutes	0 – advise while treating		
Eyelash tint, eyebrow tint and eyebrow shape	30 minutes	0 – advise while treating		
Ear piercing	15 minutes	0 – advise while treating		

? Memory jogger

1 Give two reasons why a client may not be treated.

2 How long would you book out for a half leg wax, bikini wax and eyebrow wax?

3 Why should you book the appointment while the client is still on the telephone or with you?

Getting ready for assessment

Evidence requirements

You will be observed by your assessor on at least three occasions, two of which will cover making appointments.

What you must cover during your practical assessments

Ranges

In your candidate log book you will have a list of ranges that you must cover during your assessment. These ranges cover:

1 enquiries

2 methods of making appointments

3 appointment details.

From the range you must show that:

- you have demonstrated that you have dealt with face-to-face enquiries and telephone enquiries
- you have made appointments with a client face-to-face and by telephone
- your appointment details have covered clients, name and contact details, the service, the date, the time and the member of staff that will be carrying out the treatment or nail service.

It is good practice to cover as many ranges as possible during each assessment. This will prevent you having to take too many additional assessments because there are many ranges that you have not managed to cover.

Performance criteria

What you must demonstrate during a practical observation by your tutor:

- maintaining the reception area by keeping it clean and tidy
- keeping product displays neat, clean and tidy
- reporting low levels of stationery and retail to your supervisor
- offering clients hospitality
- attending to clients and enquiries
- recording messages and appointments accurately and **confidentially**
- showing good communication skills
- making and confirming appointments accurately.

Throughout your observations you will also need to make sure that you pay attention to health, safety and hygiene throughout, as well as presenting yourself well, so read through Unit G20 Make sure your own actions reduce risks to health and safety before any practical assessment just to refresh your memory.

Top tips ✓

- Make sure you are confident and have organised your reception pens and stationery well.
- Prepare a checklist so that it is easy to check that you have everything to hand.
- Concentrate, don't let friends distract you.
- Be immaculately dressed with a ready smile on your face.

What you must know

In order to pass this unit, you will need to gather evidence during the teaching and learning of this unit before your assessor observes your practical performance. You will gather this during class work and further study and will probably file it in a portfolio of evidence. This evidence will also be signed off in your candidate log book which you will be given by your assessor. This will be an official record to show that you have covered what you need to.

 Salon life

Sunita rushed into the salon, ten minutes late. Her bus had failed to arrive on time again.

It was Sunita's turn on reception today, and she hated it. She walked past two clients who were already waiting and dumped her handbag on the desk. Then she took out her make-up bag. She wanted to put her make-up on before her boss saw her. She was glad that no one caught her doing this. She eyed one of the women in the waiting area who was huffing and tutting. Sunita became annoyed. She always seemed to get lumbered with the awkward clients.

Janie, the head therapist, came into reception. She went straight to Sunita and told her off for not letting her know that her client had arrived. Sunita rolled her eyes – it was going to be one of those days. The phone rang. Sunita lifted the receiver but replaced it straight away, as she was not yet organised. She still needed to change into her uniform, put her bag in her locker and make a coffee to wake herself up.

Sunita went through to the staff room, where she chatted and giggled for a few minutes about the party she went to last night. Then she sorted herself out.

Sunita's day soon went from bad to worse. The salon manager called her into her office and gave her an oral warning about her conduct and attitude. She said that she was responsible for therapists starting treatments late, make-up on the appointment sheets and a theft in reception. To Sunita, this was terribly unfair. She was always the person who was blamed when anything went wrong. She decided that she would start looking for another job.

List the things that Sunita did wrong.

Comment on her attitude. Was it acceptable?

How could Sunita improve her morning routine and make herself a more popular staff member?

UNIT B2

Assist with facial skin care treatments

Facial skin goes through many changes over the years. Our faces are under constant pressure from the weather and dirt in the environment, and also undergo a natural ageing process. Only some of us are lucky enough to have a naturally clear complexion that will not become too lined as we get older. We can cover up other parts of our body if they are less than perfect, but this is not so with our faces. Our faces are on show all the time and it is therefore important that we look after them. Nothing beats regular facials when it comes to keeping our skin glowing and healthy. Facial treatments are essential for thorough cleansing of the skin and increased cell renewal.

In this unit you will learn how to assist with facial skin care treatments. You will also learn how to prepare for treatments and about ways to improve the skin through the correct use of skin care products. At all times during facial skin care treatments you will also need to follow effective health, safety and hygiene procedures.

In this unit you will learn how to:

- Maintain safe and effective methods of working when assisting with facial treatments
- Consult, plan and prepare for treatments with clients
- Carry out facial treatments
- Provide aftercare advice

Here are some key terms you will meet in this unit:

Complexion – skin tone, texture and colour

Contra-actions – unwanted reactions to a treatment

Pores – tiny openings in the skin that produce oil to moisturise the skin

Effleurage – to flow, so these are stroking, smooth massage movements

Comedone extractor – a tool for blackhead removal

Petrissage – to knead, so these are circling, kneading massage movements

Rehydrate – add water or moisture

Moisturise – soften and rehydrate by the use of creams

Eczema – a dry skin condition that shows up as rough, flaky skin

Tapotement – a stimulating form of massage using cupping or pinching movements

Astringent – strong solution to cleanse the skin

Contra-indication – a condition that makes the client unsuitable for treatment such as skin infections or high blood pressure

Dehydration – lacking in water

Allergies – reactions, sensitivity

Client consultation – question-and-answer sessions with a client that are designed to find out information about them

Blemishes – skin marks

Conjunctivitis – an eye infection

Maintain safe and effective methods of working when assisting with facial treatments (1)

As with all beauty therapies, skin care treatments involve close work with the client and require close attention from you. Safe working practices are very important and you must make sure you follow much higher standards of hygiene than you might ever think of doing at home. You should also know that some facial treatments use electrical equipment, and therefore when you are assisting a therapist you need to be able to recognise safe working methods and follow instructions from the therapist.

The work area

Many different products, tools and pieces of equipment are needed for a facial treatment and you will need to set up your work area with these items before you bring your client to the treatment room. These items are listed and explained on pages 98–101.

The most important thing to remember is that when carrying out or assisting with a facial treatment, you need to be both safe and effective. This means that your work area must always be:

- organised – nothing forgotten, all equipment and tools on a trolley, set up in the order of when it will be used
- easy to reach – you will not have to overstretch to reach it or walk across the room
- hygienic – everything cleaned, disinfected and sterilised, and your couch or chair has a protective cover.

Good organisation with careful consideration of your client's needs is the key to successful preparation and a well thought out workspace for skin care treatments.

≫ Get up and go!

Take two or three photographs of work area set-ups using your mobile phone or digital camera. Upload them to a computer and see how many mistakes there are and which is the best prepared work area. Discuss your findings with your group. You could also insert the photos in a PowerPoint presentation so it is easy for the whole group to look at and make comments on.

Sterilisation and cleaning of skin care tools and equipment

As for any salon treatment, you need to maintain accepted industry hygiene practices throughout a facial treatment. Following the correct hygiene methods will prevent cross-infection, which is when germs or bacteria are transferred from one person to other, sometimes with nasty results such as skin and eye infections.

Unit G20 explains in detail how germs and bacteria can be passed on during treatments and what you should do to prevent this from happening, so refer back to pages 20–21. The table below shows how cross-infection could occur during a facial treatment and will help you to understand what hygiene means in practical terms for this particular treatment.

Stage of the facial treatment	Unhygienic practices that could lead to cross-infection
Preparing to treat the client and/or during the whole of the treatment	Completing a treatment on one client and then carrying straight on to the next client without washing your hands, or going to the toilet during the treatment and returning to the client without washing your hands
Removing blackheads	Not sterilising the blackhead extractor
Applying a mask	Not washing and sterilising the mask brush
Applying **moisturiser**	Using your fingers instead of a disposable spatula to scoop out the cream from the pot, meaning that after a few treatments the cream is full of germs from different clients

Facial treatments use quite a lot of disposable products such as cotton wool, tissues, spatulas, mask sponges, orange sticks and couch roll. Non-disposable items need to be prepared carefully for use.

- Equipment such as steamers, trolleys and magnifying lamps should be wiped over with disinfectant before and after use and metal tools such as blackhead extractors need to be sterilised.

- Mask brushes should be washed in warm soapy water, left to air dry and then placed in an ultraviolet cabinet.

- All skincare products should be removed from their containers using a spatula or orange stick.

 Top tip

Do not scoop out creams with your fingers, as this contaminates the whole pot. Always use a clean spatula.

Maintain safe and effective methods of working when assisting with facial treatments (2)

Maintaining hygiene throughout

Hygiene is not something that you only need to think about before beginning a treatment. Throughout any treatment, you must ensure that you maintain the same high standards. This applies to the tools, equipment and products that you use, and also to your own personal hygiene. Remember the following rules.

- If you sneeze or cough you must cover your mouth and turn away from the client and then go and wash your hands.
- If you blow your nose, wash your hands.
- Don't put fingers in pots and containers.
- Keep your work area tidy.
- Throw away used tissues and cotton wool immediately in a nearby foot pedal bin.

> **» Get up and go!**
>
> Make a checklist of how your skin and make-up should look so that a client will not be put off, but will instead feel confident that she is being treated by a person who knows what she is doing.

Leaving the work area clean and tidy

Remember that a tidy and clean work area is not only important for health and safety, it also shows that the salon is professional and run properly. A dirty, untidy room is an instant turn-off for any client because it demonstrates a lack of care and hygiene. After you have finished the treatment and your client has left, you must clear away all of your tools and equipment to leave your work area clean and tidy and ready for the next client. This will include:

- wiping over trolleys, couches, bins and stools with disinfectant
- washing facial tools and equipment
- putting bedding in to be laundered.

Posture and positioning while working

For you to be able to carry out a professional treatment and for the treatment to be enjoyable for the client, it is important that you are both comfortable.

A facial treatment is typically carried out while the client lies on a comfortable couch. The client may lie completely flat or semi-inclined and must be positioned comfortably. Your client should be able to remain relaxed during the treatment without having to twist or move so that you can reach her.

For you, bad posture will cause physical aches and pains. In addition, the treatment will probably not be as good because it has been carried out in an awkward position.

You will need to decide whether you will stand or sit behind the couch. It depends on:

- the height and angle of the couch – whether it is flat or sloping
- your height and whether you can reach the client if you sit down.

Adjust the height of the couch so that you don't have to reach too far up or down, and make sure that all the equipment and tools you need are within easy reach. It is very important that you do not overstretch your neck and back to reach tools or the client's face because you will end up with a long-term back problem. Overstretching will also affect the muscles and veins in your legs and could possibly cause varicose veins over time.

Top tip

When standing for long periods of time, move a little to keep the circulation going. For example, every now and then:

- move from one foot to the other
- bend the knee back a few times, then repeat on the other foot.

Environmental conditions

Lighting
Lighting must be bright and clear for the skin inspection, but soft and relaxing for the rest of the facial treatment. A light that can be dimmed is ideal, along with a magnifying lamp for inspection work.

Ambience
This means the atmosphere or mood that is created within the treatment room or salon. This is important because the aim is to get the client to relax and enjoy her treatment and the whole experience.

Relaxing music, pleasant-smelling oils and scented candles can all act to create a favourable atmosphere.

Heating and ventilation
The facial treatment area needs to be warm and inviting. It is usual during a facial for a client to become cold. This is because when they relax their body temperature can drop. For this reason it is necessary to have covers that can be placed on the client, such as a blanket or duvet, as well as keeping the temperature of the room fairly warm. Thermostatically controlled central heating is the best, as heaters that you need to turn on and off when needed are not very efficient.

Inspect the client's skin under a bright light

? Memory jogger

1 What sort of lighting is needed to carry out facial treatments?
2 Why is posture important when carrying out a treatment?
3 How can relaxing affect a client's temperature?
4 What is the best form of heating in a treatment room?

Consult, plan and prepare for treatments with clients [1]

Before beginning any skin care treatment, you need to make sure that both you and the client are well prepared. You will need to chat to your client about why she would like a facial, record the client's contact details and information about her skin and her home skin care routine, and carry out a simple analysis to help you to decide the skin type, identify any problems and be able to plan a treatment suitable for the client.

However, the first step before collecting your client and bringing her to the treatment room is to set up your work area with all the materials that you will need. These are:

- basics – the disposable products, laundry and workspace requirements
- tech tools – the tools, such as tweezers and scissors, that you will need
- products – all the creams and lotions needed for the treatment.

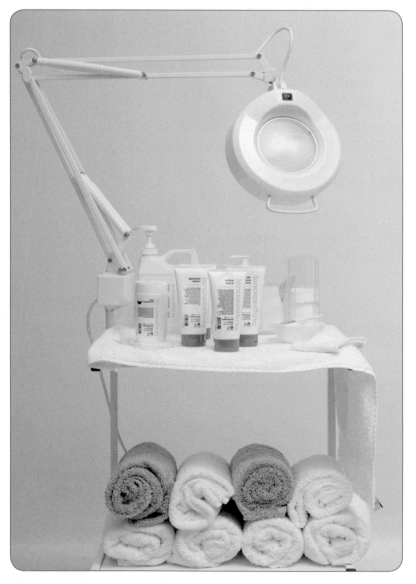

What you need to carry out a facial skin care treatment

Basics

When setting up for a facial skin care treatment, make sure you have all the basics to hand.

Item	Purpose
Dampened cotton wool	Cotton wool squares: for removing cleanser and putting on toner. They need to be large enough to wrap around your first two fingers.
	Cotton wool half moons: these are placed under the bottom eyelashes, to protect the skin under the eyes from the make-up that is being cleaned off.
	Eye pads (circles or squares): these rest on the eye while using the magnifying lamp for skin inspection or blackhead removal. They can be soaked in witch hazel to soothe the eyes while the client is wearing a face mask.
Dry cotton wool	To cover the tip of an orange stick for removing eye make-up.
Split tissues	To blot excess toner or moisturiser. Tissues are normally two-ply – this means that each tissue is made up of two very thin layers. For the purpose of beauty treatments, however, tissues are split as this makes them more economical to use and easier to curve around the shape of the face.
Sponges	These can be used with warm water to remove mask products from the skin. However, they are not easy to clean and sterilise. They need to be washed in very hot soapy water, dried thoroughly and then placed in an ultraviolet sterilising cabinet. The other option is for a salon to charge enough for a facial so that the sponge can be given to the client at the end of her treatment. Otherwise, it is best to use damp cotton wool squares for mask removal.
Towels	You will need one hand towel to dry your own hands during the treatment, one medium-sized towel for placing across the client's chest, and one large towel for covering her body during the treatment (if a blanket is not used).
Blanket	In the winter months, a honeycomb blanket may be needed to keep the client warm during the treatment.
Fitted couch sheet	To protect the couch from marks and product spills during a treatment.
Couch roll	This is used to cover the fitted couch sheet so that it does not need to be washed after each treatment. It is also used to protect the towel lying over the client's chest, and the pillow and the headband from skin care and mask products.
Headband or turban	This is used to protect the client's hair from the products and to prevent her hair from getting in the way of the treatment.
Gown	As the client needs to remove her top clothing, you may need to give her a gown to wear to prevent any embarrassment.
Waste bin	A pedal bin with a lid is best for hygiene purposes, as you can open it without touching it with your hands.
Sterilising jar	This should be filled with antiseptic or disinfectant solution, so that small metal tools such as blackhead extractors and tweezers can be placed in it during the treatment. The solution will help to keep germ levels down, but it will not destroy germs completely. The solution should be changed after every client.
Dishes	Small plastic or metal dishes are needed to hold cotton wool and tissues, as well as the client's jewellery.

 Top tip

How to prepare dampened cotton wool squares:

- Cut squares approximately 80 cm^2 in size from a cotton wool roll.
- Take about four to six squares and hold them between the palms of your hands under a running tap. When they are soaked through, squeeze out the water so that they are only damp and not dripping.
- Peel back thin layers from your thick pad of cotton wool. You should have about 16–20 pads. These are your facial pads for removing and applying products.

 Top tip

Each salon has its own way of preparing a client for a treatment, so you will need to find out how your workplace sets up, for example, whether they use sheets and blankets, or towels.

Consult, plan and prepare for treatments with clients (2)

Potions

When setting up for a facial skin care treatment, you need to make sure that you have different types of products to suit different skin types. You will learn how to determine a client's skin type on page 106.

Product	Purpose	Types
Eye make-up remover	These are mild cleansing products that dissolve eye make-up so that it can be easily wiped off without rubbing the eyes.	Eye make-up remover is available as an oil, lotion or gel. Some remove waterproof make-up.
Cleansers	To remove old make-up. To clean dirt, dust and grime from the skin and **pores**. To remove oil and dead skin cells.	Cream – this thick, creamy cleanser is used for dry or mature skin types. It dissolves make-up quickly. Milk – this is a thin, runny cleanser that can be used on most skin types except very dry skin. It is ideal for young or normal skin types, but is not very good at removing heavy or waterproof make-up. Lotion – this is similar in thickness to a milk cleanser but includes ingredients to help spotty and combination skins, which are usually found in younger clients. Facial washes – these can be liquids, gels or lotions. They are gently rubbed into the skin with some water to make a lather. Facial washes can be used on any skin as long as moisturiser is applied afterwards, as the skin can feel quite tight. Facial washes are especially good for men and people who like to feel freshly washed.
Toners	To remove any left-over cleanser from the skin. To dissolve oil. To refresh and cool the skin. To tighten the skin and **pores**.	Toners come in different strengths and are chosen depending on the skin type. The main ingredients are water, alcohol, colour and perfume. The greater the alcohol content, the stronger the toner. Toners for oily problem skins are called **astringents** and have the highest alcohol content.
Face masks*	Face masks are usually applied towards the end of a facial, after the skin has been cleansed, steamed and massaged. A mask should never be applied to skin that has not been thoroughly cleansed. Depending on the ingredients, face masks can: • deep clean the skin and **pores** • remove oil and dead skin cells • deeply **moisturise** and nourish the skin • tighten the pores • soften fine lines • soothe sensitive skins.	Setting – these masks are usually made of clay powder. They are mixed with distilled water or toner to make a paste that can be painted on the skin with a mask brush. Non-setting – these masks can be creams or gels in a tube or pot. Specialised – these are nourishing warm oil masks or deeply moisturising paraffin wax masks. Food – just as the name says, these face masks can be made using ingredients from your own fridge at home.
Moisturisers	To soften and protect the skin's surface. To **rehydrate** the skin. To help the application of make-up by providing a smooth base.	As with cleansers, moisturisers can be: • creams for dry skins • lotions for oily skins • milks for young, normal or sensitive skins.

* For Level 1 you only need to know how to use a ready-made non-setting face mask. However, it is helpful if you have a basic knowledge of the other types that you might see being used in the salon.

>> **Get up and go!**

Try out these recipes for food masks.

For dry skin

Mash avocado, add egg yolk and mix until creamy. Apply to the face with a spatula. Leave for 10–15 minutes, then rinse off.

For oily skin

Mix oatmeal and honey together, then apply to the face with a spatula. Leave for 10–15 minutes, then rinse off.

When using food ingredients, you should use the masks as soon as you have made them, as they can go off very quickly. Only use eggs with the Lion mark.

Tech tools

When setting up for a facial skin care treatment, you need to prepare all the tools you will need.

Item	Purpose
Spatula	A spatula is a wide wooden stick that is used to scoop out cream or lotion from pots. Fingers should never be used, as this is very unhygienic and could result in cross-infection. A spatula is also used to tuck the client's hair into a headband instead of your fingers.
Orange sticks	These are made of orange wood, which is slightly bendy. One end is pointed and the other end is shaped like a hoof. Both ends of the orange stick are coated in cotton wool for hygiene purposes, as the cotton wool can be removed and thrown away after use. The cotton wool softens the tip for safety when cleaning around the eyes.
Comedone extractor	This loop-end tool is designed to remove blackheads. It is pressed onto a blackhead, then steady, gentle pressure is applied. If the blackhead is ready, its contents will pop out.
Mask brush	This is usually a strong bristle brush that is used to paint the mask on to the skin. Some brushes are fan shaped. They are very hard to sterilise completely, so care must be taken to wash them thoroughly with hot soapy water, leave them to dry and then place them in an ultraviolet sterilising cabinet for the recommended time. Alternatively, a disposable spatula can be used to apply some masks.

[?] **Memory jogger**

1 Moisturisers are used to:

A Hydrate the skin

B Tone the skin

C Wash the skin

D Exfoliate the skin

2 Give three types of face masks that can be used.

3 The best type of cleanser for oily to combination skins is:

A Milk

B Lotion

C Cream

D Facial wash

4 How does eye make-up remover work to remove eye make-up?

5 List three tech tools that you will need to set up for a facial.

Consult, plan and prepare for treatments with clients (3)

Client consultation

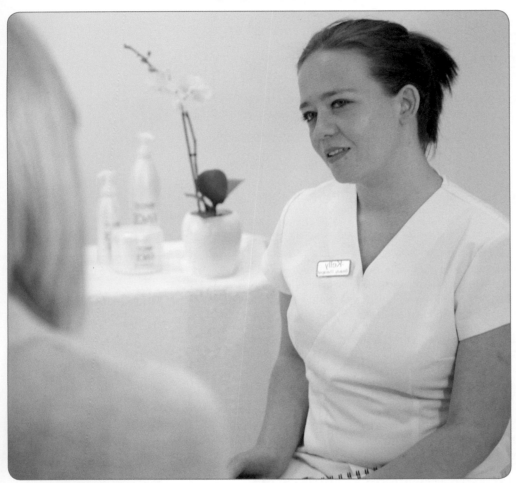

Carrying out a **client consultation**

Planning and preparing your treatment will always involve a **client consultation**. Until you have talked to the client about why she has come to the salon for a facial and assessed her skin type and any problems, it will not be possible for you to decide which products and techniques to use on your client. Client consultation involves the following three methods:

- questioning and recording information
- visual analysis
- manual analysis – this is when you feel the smoothness, softness, firmness and hydration of the client's skin.

Questioning

Clients will want facials for many different reasons. Depending on their reasons, this will help to shape the type of facial that should be offered to them and the techniques used.

Top tip ✓

At first you will watch and learn from the therapist while she is carrying out a consultation. Eventually you will have gained enough experience to carry out the consultation yourself under the supervision of the therapist.

For relaxation and a feeling of well-being	To add moisture to dry or **dehydrated** skin
Reasons why a client might want a facial	
To help clear spots and **blemishes**	To reduce the oil on greasy skin

Reasons for a facial treatment

It is therefore very important that you ask the client about her wishes and needs from the facial and listen and respond carefully. Sitting down to talk with the client about what she wants will also give you the opportunity to ask her about her skin and any problem areas, as well as the skin care routine that she follows at home.

FACIAL CONSULTATION CARD

DATE 12/02/10   CLIENT'S NAME Miss Nadia Shah

ADDRESS 14 Willow Crescent, Newtown N01 3JA   DATE OF BIRTH 26/08/78

TELEPHONE NUMBER (H) 0208 976 1133   (W) 0207 612 1060

CONDITION OF SKIN ON INSPECTION

Clear complexion, fine lines around the eyes, a few broken capillaries on cheek area. Feels slightly dry.

CONTRA-INDICATIONS/CONDITIONS

No contra-indications. Comedones around nose and chin.

PRODUCTS USED

Nourishing Nature's range for dry skin.

HOMECARE ADVICE

Drink more water to rehydrate the skin.
Use sunscreen and exfoliate weekly.

PRODUCT SALES

Nourishing Nature's trial pack for dry skin.

COMMENTS

Client was very relaxed and pleased with how her skin felt. Has re-booked for a month's time.

CLIENT SIGNATURE

RECORD OF TREATMENTS

DATE	TREATMENT	THERAPIST
12/02/10	Facial	Sarah Walker

A typical consultation card for a facial treatment

While you question the client, you need to start filling in a **client consultation** card with the information that the client gives you. An example of a consultation card for a facial skin care treatment is shown above. Some of the information will be filled in later, after you have studied the skin, and some when you have completed the treatment, but all of the information you need is included in the diagram on page 104 for easy reference. Have a look at Unit B1 Prepare and maintain salon treatment work areas to refresh your memory about why it is important to record the information.

» Get up and go!

Design a simple flow chart showing the stages of the consultation that you can use to jog your memory. Display it on a postcard so that it will fit on your trolley next to you. Remember to laminate it so that you protect it from spills and splashes.

Consult, plan and prepare for treatments with clients (4)

Recording information

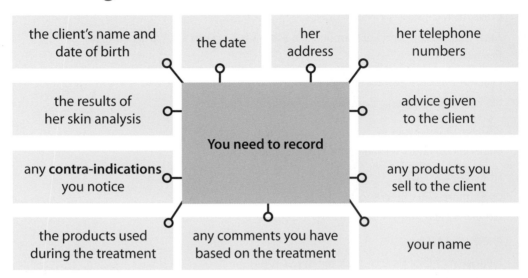

Information you need to record for a facial skin care treatment

 Top tips

- Name – there could be two clients with the same surname, so to avoid confusion, make sure you always write down both the client's first name and surname.
- Address – remember to include the postcode.
- Telephone number – one telephone number is not enough. If you need to call a client at short notice to tell her that you have to cancel her appointment and you have her home phone number but she is at work, you will not be able to get in touch, so always ask for a home number and a work or mobile number.
- Date of birth – you may need to find out your client's date of birth, as if she is under the age of 16 a parent or guardian must be present throughout the treatment. Also the parent or guardian must sign the consultation to agree for the treatment to go ahead – this is called giving consent.

Visual analysis

After talking to the client and noting down the information you need to record, you then need to study the client's skin visually. This should be done in good light so that you are able to see the skin's condition and texture and includes finding out about:

- skin type
- skin condition
- **contra-indications**.

Skin types and conditions

Deciding on a client's skin type is essential before you can decide on the best treatment for her skin. There are four main skin types, and each of the four skin types may also have other characteristics that are important for you to note.

The four main skin types

Characteristics that each of the four skin types may display

> ## >> Get up and go!
>
> Make some key cards to help you remember the different types of skin and the characteristics of each. Write 'normal skin' on one card, then turn it over and write a description of the characteristics of normal skin on the back. Make a card like this for each of the skin types. You can use these to test each other on skin types and conditions.

> ## ? Memory jogger
>
> 1 What are the three types of consultation techniques?
> 2 List four pieces of information that you would need to record when carrying out a consultation.
> 3 Why is it important to ask a client about her wishes?

Consult, plan and prepare for treatments with clients (5)

Deciding on a client's skin type is not always a simple process – it can take several years to master each part of a facial treatment and become an expert. However, for Level 1 only background knowledge of the basics is required. Let's take a closer look at skin types.

Skin types

Normal skin

Normal skin is a rare skin type. It is usually found in children and young clients. It is smooth and clear with no **blemishes**. It feels soft to touch and has very tiny **pores** that are difficult to see. This type of skin needs lots of gentle care to keep it normal.

Oily skin

Oily skin is caused when too much oil is produced in the skin. Although we need oil to keep the skin smooth, when the body produces too much oil this causes problems. Oily skin has a shiny **complexion** with lots of blackheads and **blemishes**. The **pores** are quite large and the skin can be quite thick. An oily skin can start or become worse as a teenager, when puberty hormones are most active.

Dry skin

Dry skin is lacking in oil and may flake and chap easily. It can feel tight after washing, especially if soap is used. Dry skin absorbs creams and lotions quickly, and can become lined and wrinkled early (especially around the eyes) unless it is moisturised well. Poor diet or **dehydration** can cause dry skin or make it worse.

Combination skin

Combination skin is made up of two skin types. These types vary but the most common is normal or dry skin on the cheek area, and an oily part on the nose and chin, and across the forehead (known as the T-zone). The oily T-zone shows up as a shiny nose, chin and forehead with blackheads.

> **» Get up and go!**
>
> What skin type are you?
>
> Take a close look at your skin in the mirror. Use a good light and decide what skin type you have.
>
> Next, pair up with a friend and inspect each other's skin. Did you both agree on the skin type?

Contra-indications

A **contra-indication** is a condition that makes or could make a client unsuitable for a treatment. At Level 1 you are not responsible for deciding whether or not a client has a contra-indication, but you must be aware of them and be able to recognise the signs so that you can tell a senior therapist if you notice anything unusual.

Whatever level of experience therapists have, they are not qualified to diagnose medical conditions. Quite often during your treatments you may have an idea of what medical condition a client may have, but you must refer them to their GP. You must also make sure that you do not cause the client alarm or embarrassment by talking loudly about a contra-indication so that other people may hear or in a way that may worry the client.

Working around contra-indications

Some contra-indications can be worked around and you can adapt your treatment in line with the client's needs. Usually you will avoid the area that must not be worked on, but sometimes it is difficult to do this and so you may need to:

- cover the area with a plaster
- cover the area with barrier cream.

Contra-indications that may be worked around include:

- non-infectious conditions
- non-recent scar tissue (over six months old)
- mild bruising
- grazes or small cuts.

Skin disorders that may restrict treatment include:

- healed **eczema** – this will present as very dry and parched skin and can quite often look very lined
- psoriasis – this is scaly flakes of skin, quite often red and inflamed. It is best to completely avoid these areas as the products and procedures could cause further inflammation
- redness – adapt your methods, for example use gentle products and don't carry out stimulating massage movements
- bruising – work around the bruising so that you don't cause pain to the client
- skin irritation – it is recommended that you postpone the treatment until the irritation goes as it could be a sign of an allergy.

Consult, plan and prepare for treatments with clients (6)

Total contra-indications

Some **contra-indications** could be made worse by treatment or could be infectious and spread to you and your other clients. These are called total contra-indications. You must never treat a client who has a total contra-indication.

You will need to look out for:

- splits or blisters around the nose and mouth that could be a cold sore
- bloodshot and watery eyes that could be an allergy or **conjunctivitis**
- extremely red skin – it could be a sign of an allergy or an injury
- swelling or lumps – it could just be bruising but could also be something much more serious that needs to be checked by a GP.

The following photos should help you to know what to look out for when you check a client's skin for contra-indications.

Skin infections such as impetigo

Cold sores

Conjunctivitis

Bruising

Scar tissue less than six months old

Recent sunburn

Cuts and grazes

Eczema

Allergies

Some clients may be allergic to certain ingredients contained in products. You should always ask your client if she has any known **allergies** and check the list of ingredients on the label of the products you are planning to use.

It may be that you check for allergies beforehand but a client nevertheless reacts badly to a product by showing one of these signs: itching, tightness, blistering, watery eyes, excess sweating, swelling or redness. If this happens you must take steps to remove the product immediately and tell your supervisor, who will advise you and the client on what should be done. She may be advised to bathe the area with cool water and see her GP.

 Top tip

If you notice anything unusual on the skin, always ask your tutor or senior therapist to check for you before you start the treatment.

Consult, plan and prepare for treatments with clients (7)

Adapting your manner for different clients

Although your manner must always be professional, your consultation with your client gives you the opportunity to find out what your client is like. Remember that the conversation and personality that one client may enjoy, another may not. Find out:

- what your client likes and does not like
- what your client's personality is like; for example, shy or extrovert
- whether your client is talkative or quiet.

As an assistant therapist you do not yet have the client experience that more qualified therapists have and so it is important that you try to develop people skills and learn how and when you need to adapt your body language, speech and manner. Use this consultation time to learn about the client so that you can adapt your style of communication as well as the treatment.

Preparing the client

Once you have finished the **client consultation**, you need to get the client ready for her facial treatment.

1 Ask the client to remove any jewellery she is wearing and ask her to store it safely.

2 Ask the client to remove the clothes from her top half, and take them and hang them up. If she has to go to a treatment cubicle to change, you will need to give her a gown to wear to prevent any embarrassment.

3 Help the client on to the couch. Remove the gown and cover the client with the blankets or towels, and ask her if she is warm and comfortable.

4 Protect the client's hair with a headband. Tuck either tissue or couch roll under the headband to keep it as clean as possible. Place a medium-sized towel across the client's chest, then slip her bra straps down over her upper arms and tuck the towel over and under the straps, to protect them from the products.

 Top tip

If a client removes her jewellery and does place it in a dish, the jewellery dish should then be placed on top of the trolley so that the client is able to see it at all times. This is for security reasons and it also acts as a memory jogger, so that the client does not forget her jewellery when she leaves.

Consulting, planning and preparing for treatments with clients: a checklist

1 Have you prepared yourself and checked your personal presentation?

2 Have you set up your workplace and checked that you have what you need and that your equipment and tools are organised, easy to reach and properly sterilised or disinfected?

3 Have you removed your watch and jewellery?

4 Have you washed your hands?

5 Have you carried out the consultation?

6 Have you assessed the condition of your client's skin?

7 Have you checked for **contra-indications**?

8 Have you asked the client to remove her jewellery?

9 Have you asked the client to remove the clothes from her top half, helped her on to the couch, covered her, protected her hair and bra straps and checked if she is warm and comfortable?

If so, you are ready to begin the facial treatment.

 Salon life

Deepak started to cleanse the skin of his client but she started to wriggle and complained that it was stinging a bit. Deepak though that this would be fine and they agreed he would carry on, so he then toned the skin, but he could see the skin getting redder and redder and his client's lips then began to swell too. His supervisor had popped out for a ten-minute break to get a bite to eat, so he did not have anyone to ask what to do. He checked the record card and there was no information to say that his client had an allergy, so he removed the cleanser and toner that he had used with cool water and tried to calm the reaction with different products. The condition got worse and by the time his supervisor returned the client's face was very red and swollen and his supervisor was horrified.

Was it Deepak's fault?

What could Deepak have done to lessen the problem?

What could you do to prevent this happening to you?

? Memory jogger

1 List three contra-indications that you could work around.

2 List three contra-indications that will prevent you carrying out the treatment.

3 List the steps you need to take to prepare your client.

4 List three signs of an allergy.

5 How do you protect a contra-indication that you can work around?

Carry out facial treatments (1)

A facial should be relaxing and enjoyable for the client, as well as being beneficial to her skin. Learning about carrying out a facial involves learning about several smaller treatments that are carried out to:

- deep clean the **pores**
- nourish and **rehydrate** the skin
- relax the muscles
- improve the circulation
- brighten the **complexion**.

After a facial, the client should feel relaxed and her skin should glow.

Step-by-step facial

There are many steps involved in a facial skin care treatment. Before we go into them in detail, it will help to look at this summary so that the procedure is clear.

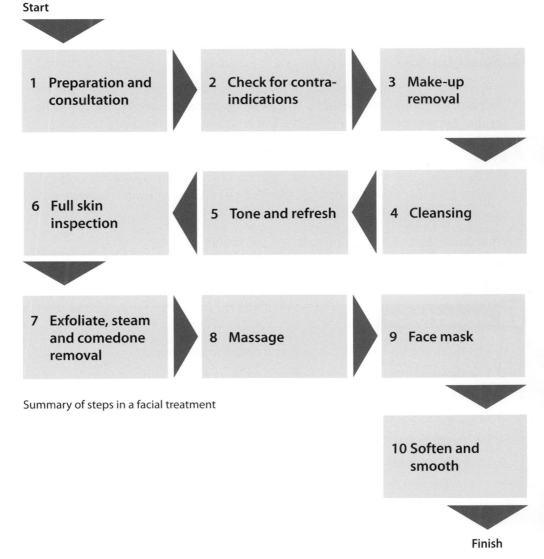

Summary of steps in a facial treatment

Top tip

Throughout the facial, explain what you are doing and why. This will reassure the client and help her to relax and enjoy it.

Make-up removal

When your client is prepared for her facial and comfortably positioned on the couch, the first thing you need to do is to remove any make-up that she might be wearing. This is shown on page 116.

 Top tip

You may need to repeat the eye make-up removal process for very heavy or waterproof make-up.

Cleansing

Your next step is to cleanse the client's face. Choose an appropriate cleanser for the client – look back at page 100 to remind yourself of the different types of cleansers available.

The cleansing routine is carried out with massage movements. Massage has three main movements.

- **Effleurage**: this is a gentle stroking movement used at the beginning or end of the treatment or to join up other movements. It has a soothing and relaxing effect. This is the technique used for cleansing.
- **Petrissage**: these movements are circular or kneading movements. The hands, thumbs or fingertips are used to apply pressure to the muscles by lifting, rolling and pushing.
- **Tapotement**: this is a more stimulating movement in which the fingers, sides or palms of the hands produce light tapping, quick pinching or gentle slapping movements.

For Level 1, it is not necessary for you to follow a set massage routine using all the movements. However, it is important to carry out some sort of pattern that is relaxing to the client. The photos on pages 116–120 illustrate a simple cleansing routine for you to follow.

All movements are done lightly and your hands must never leave the client's skin.

Tone and refresh

After cleansing the client's skin twice, you then need refresh her skin and remove the last traces of cleanser using a toning lotion. This is shown on page 121.

 Top tip

Remember that you will have to write down the products you use on the client's face on her record card.

Carry out facial treatments (2)

Step-by-step facial

Full skin inspection

When your client's skin is completely clean, dry and grease-free, your senior therapist will carry out a thorough skin inspection under the magnifying lamp. It is only now when the skin is absolutely clean that you and your senior therapist will be able to see the true skin type, any disorders and make a final check for any **contra-indications**. You will then also be able to plan the rest of your facial deciding:

- on the products to be used
- on the type of face mask
- whether you need to slightly change your treatment plan.

When carrying out the skin inspection, make notes on the record card.

Skin disorders and contra-indications

Look out for signs of these, which were covered on pages 107–109.

Skin colour • Does it have a healthy glow? • Are there areas of redness that could suggest sensitivity? • Is the skin tanned or is it a yellowy colour?	**The eyes** • Are there laughter lines around the eyes? • Are there dark circles or puffiness around or under the eyes?
Skin texture Touch the skin. How does it feel? • Soft or rough? • Dry or oily? • Flaky or smooth? • Thin or thick? • Firm or loose?	**Skin and muscle tone** • Is the skin young and firm with good muscle tone and tight skin? • Is the skin around the eyes and mouth loose with lines and wrinkles? • Are there frown lines on the forehead?
The T-zone • Is the T-zone shiny with blackheads, spots and open pores?	**Client information** Ask the client: • what products she uses on her skin • what her normal skincare routine is

What to look for during a full skin inspection

» Get up and go!

Practise some massage movements on another therapist so that she can give you feedback on how to improve.

Exfoliate, steam and comedone removal, and massage

The next steps in the facial treatment are exfoliation, steaming and comedone extraction, and massage, which will all be carried out by a senior therapist.

Massage is a very skilful part of the facial treatment and can take a long time to master, so make sure that you watch the senior therapist carefully. As you become more skilled at your treatment, you may be allowed to carry out part of the massage..

Face mask

When the senior therapist has completed the massage, you will then apply the face mask. Before applying the face mask, make sure that your client's skin is free of oils and creams. Then choose a pre-prepared, non-setting mask to suit your client's skin type.

Soften and smooth

The final stage of the facial treatment is applying moisturiser to the client's skin. When you have finished, leave the client to relax for a couple of minutes, and go and wash your hands. Then offer your client a mirror, so that she can check her **complexion**.

Finishing touches

When you have finished the facial treatment, you must:

- ask your client how she feels and if she is pleased with her treatment
- give your client homecare advice (see pages 124–125)
- check the finished result with the senior therapist
- check the time, to make sure that the treatment was cost effective and carried out within an acceptable time (see page 89)
- make sure that the workplace is left tidy, clean and ready for further treatments.

Remember to complete the client's record card with as much information as possible on the products you used, the homecare advice you gave her on how to improve the condition of her skin and when to return for another salon treatment, your comments on how you and the client thought the treatment went, and the date, the type of facial and your name.

 Top tips

- It is very important to check that every trace of the mask is removed – make sure that no mask remains anywhere on the skin. Check behind the ears and under the chin.
- Always follow the manufacturer's instructions when using beauty products. The instructions should have information about:
  - how to use the product
  - how long to leave it on the skin
  - how to store it
  - how to use it safely.

» Get up and go!

Design a client feedback sheet that you can use to ask clients how they felt about their facial treatment.

Discuss the feedback with the rest of your class and your tutor.

? Memory jogger

1 At what stage in the facial do you apply the face mask?
2 Why is it important to write down on the record card all of the products that you use during a facial?
3 When do you give the client homecare advice?
4 Where on the face would the oily section usually be found with a combination skin type?
5 What would the texture of the skin feel like on a client with mature skin?
6 Why must the skin be completely clean and free of make-up before carrying out a full skin inspection?

Carry out facial treatments (3)

Step-by-step facial

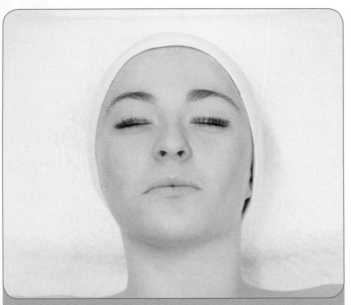

1 Make sure the client is prepared for her facial.

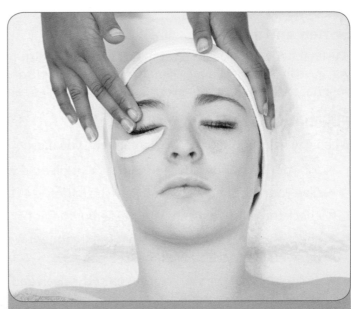

2 Place half moons under the bottom lashes and ask client to close her eyes. Squeeze a small amount of eye make-up remover on to a spatula. Dip your index finger into the cleanser and gently rub on and around the eye in a circular movement.

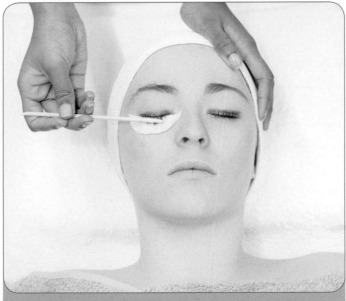

3 Using a covered orange stick, use gentle downward strokes until the eye and lashes are free from make-up and cleanser. Repeat on the other eye. Then ask the client to open her eyes so that you can clean underneath them.

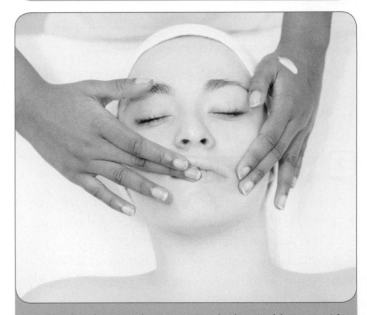

4 Gently rub some cleanser on to the lips. Hold on one side of the mouth for support, then wipe the make-up away with the other hand using damp cotton wool. Then hold the other side of the mouth, and repeat.

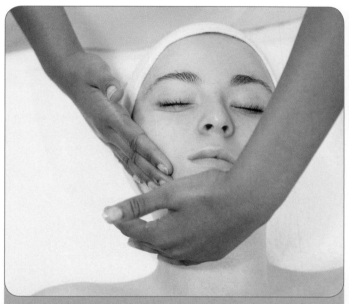

5 Squeeze a small amount of cleanser into the palm of your hands, then put your hands together so that you have the cleanser in both hands. Gently press your hands over the face and neck of your client, to coat her skin in cleanser.

6 Using gentle, upward **effleurage** strokes, distribute the cleanser evenly over the face.

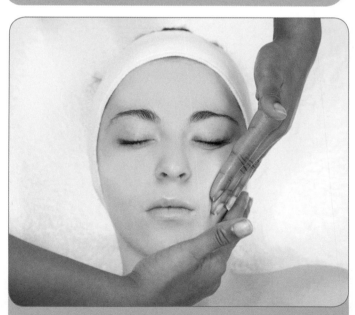

7 Following the direction of the brows, gently circle the eyes with the middle fingers to distribute the cleanser around the eyes.

8 Use gentle upward **effleurage** strokes to spread the cleanser over the cheeks.

Carry out facial treatments (4)

Step-by-step facial

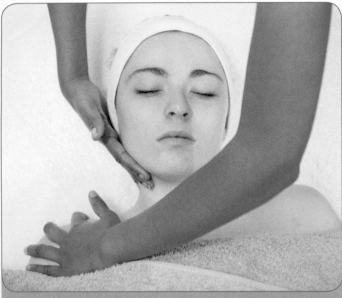

9 Using light movements, apply eight upward strokes to the client's shoulders, chest area and neck with the palms of your hands. Start with the left side and gradually work to the right side. Then repeat, this time working from the right side to the left side.

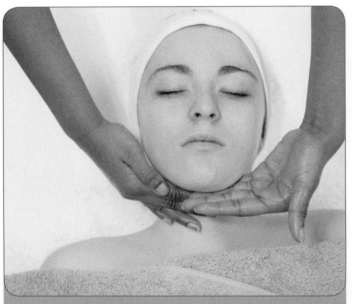

10 Apply eight upward strokes to the client's neck with the palms of your hands. Start with the left side and gradually work to the right side. Then repeat, this time working from the right side to the left side.

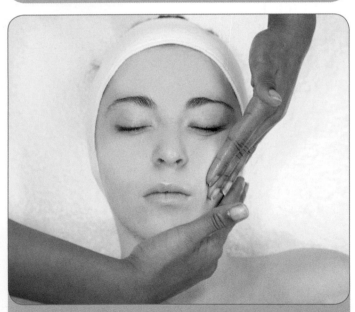

11 Using the palms of the hands, slide to the left cheek and stroke upwards eight times.

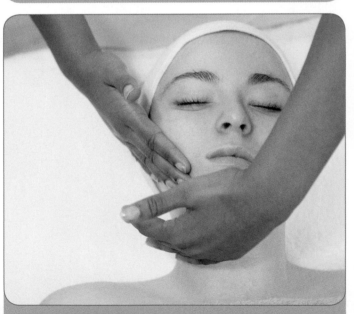

12 Slide to the right cheek and stroke upwards eight times.

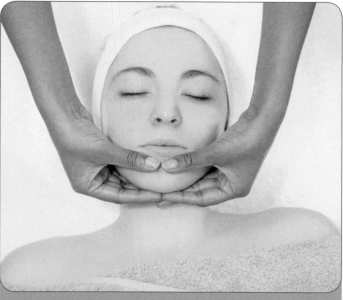

13 Slide to the chin and carry out upward thumb circles eight times.

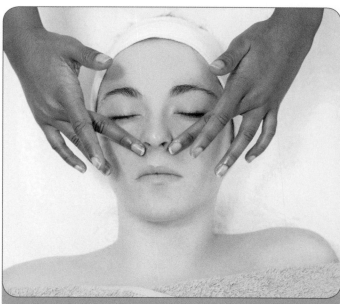

14 Using middle or index fingers, circle eight times under and around the sides of the nose.

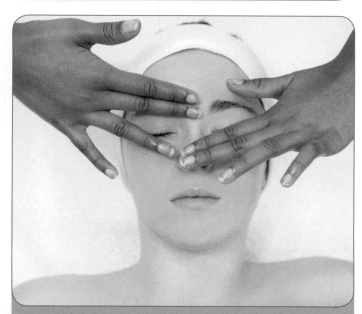

15 Slide up to the bridge of the nose and stroke upwards four times.

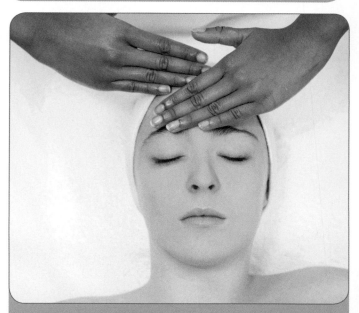

16 Slide up to the forehead and stroke upwards eight times, moving from the left to the right and then back again.

Carry out facial treatments (5)

Step-by-step facial

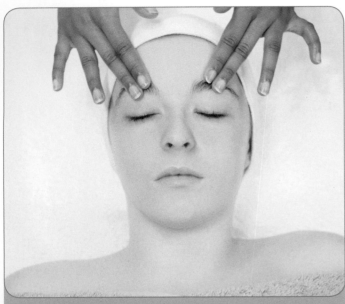

17 Slide your hands to the middle of the forehead and circle the eyes gently four times in the direction of growth of the eyebrow. Slide to the temples and apply gentle pressure to complete the cleansing routine.

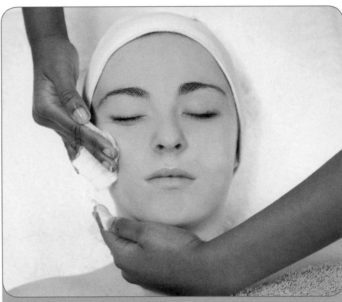

18 Take two damp cotton wool squares and wrap them around your first two fingers, and use them to remove the cleanser, which has now mixed with the dirt and face make-up. Use exactly the same strokes as for the cleansing routine (steps 9 to 17).

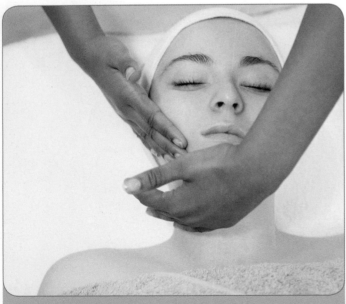

19 Carry out a second cleanse by repeating steps 5 to 19.

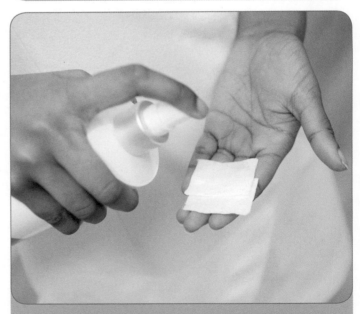

20 Take two more damp cotton wool squares and soak them in toning lotion.

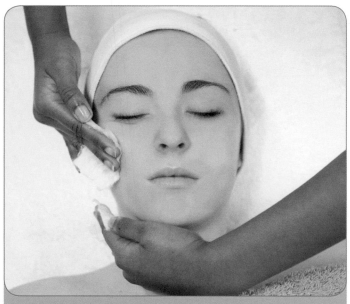

21 Wrap the cotton wool around your fingers and repeat the cleaning routine, using the toner on the cotton wool instead. This will tone the skin and remove the last traces of cleanser.

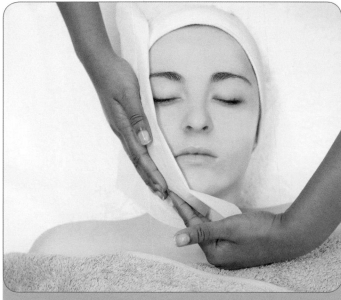

22 Using a split tissue, blot the toning lotion. Tone the skin a second time.

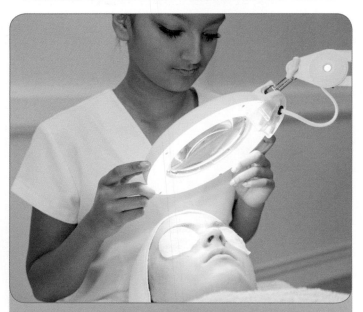

23 Carry out a skin inspection under the magnifying lamp.

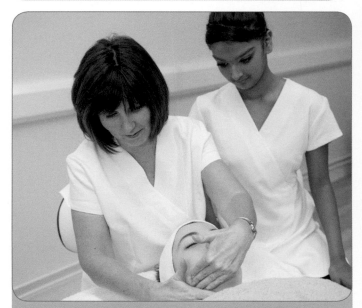

24 The senior therapist will carry out a skin exfoliating treatment, steam and comedone extraction. Tone and blot the skin by repeating steps 21 and 22. The senior therapist will then massage the client's face, neck and shoulders. The massage should last about 15–20 minutes.

Carry out facial treatments (6)

Step-by-step facial

25 Place enough mask in a bowl to coat all your client's face and neck. Using a mask brush and starting at the neck, apply the mask to the skin and move upwards evenly in smooth strokes, finishing with the forehead. Avoid the lips, eyes, nostrils and hairline.

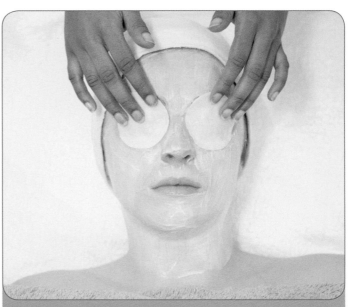

26 After the face mask has been applied, place eye circles over your client's eyes, then leave her to rest and relax for about 10 minutes, depending on the manufacturer's instructions.

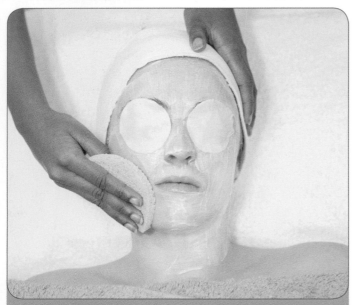

27 After 10 minutes remove the eye pads and press damp sponges over the mask, allowing the water to soak in. Starting at the neck and working up over the cheeks on to the nose and forehead, remove all the face mask with firm upward strokes.

28 Tone and blot the skin and apply moisturiser for the client's skin type using the same massage routine to apply the moisturiser as you did for the cleanser. Blot the skin if there is too much moisturiser on it.

Making sure your client enjoys her facial

A facial should be an enjoyable and relaxing treatment for your client, but this could be spoiled if you are careless or disorganised. A client may not enjoy a facial if the therapist:

- has offensive body odour or bad breath or smells of tobacco
- harms or scratches the skin with jewellery, watches or nails that are too long
- massages the skin excessively or roughly
- gets facial creams or products into the client's eyes
- breathes into the client's face
- is not hygienic or careful enough
- removes cream carelessly and incorrectly, leaving a greasy film behind the ears, under the chin or in other areas
- does not permit the client to relax, either by talking too much or being tense while giving the treatment
- is disorganised and needs to leave the client to go and fetch materials and products
- has heavy, rough or cold hands.

Take care to avoid these mistakes!

Male facials

More men are having facial treatments than ever before. It is now seen as acceptable for men to visit salons to have treatments, and there are ranges of skin care products available in shops and salons that are targeted at the male skin care market. This has become a very profitable business.

 Top tip

Although you want to make sure that your client is enjoying her treatment by asking her how it feels or if she is comfortable, asking her too many times during the facial can ruin the atmosphere of the treatment and mean that it will not be as relaxing for her. Try not to question her more than a couple of times.

 Get up and go!

Visit some local salons and find out about the male skin care treatments on offer. How do they differ from a female skin care treatment?

 Salon life

During a consultation, Petra asked her client what she hoped to gain from her facial. The client said that she had a big dinner party that evening and wanted to go out feeling like a 'new woman'. The client said that her skin was dry and flaky, and that her make-up wouldn't go on very smoothly. The client hoped that Petra would be able to improve the texture of her skin, so that her make-up would look great for the party.

It was obvious to Petra that the client had not been advised as to what a facial is, and therefore had her heart set on:

- a treatment for dry flaky skin
- being able to apply great make-up for her dinner party.
  1. How could Petra explain the purpose of a facial to her client?
  2. What other choices could Petra give her client?

Write down or discuss how you would deal with these problems.

Provide aftercare advice

So that the beneficial effects of the facial treatment lasts, it is important to give the client some advice after the treatment.

You should advise your client that the recommended interval between facial treatments is one month in order to keep the skin in great condition. This also gives your client the opportunity to book a further appointment with the salon.

The facial treatment has given your client's skin a boost. After the treatment, her skin will enjoy better circulation and a softer texture, and should be the cleanest it has been for a while. It is therefore important to give your client follow-up advice, so that she can experience the long-term benefits of her treatment. The table below details the follow-up advice that you should give.

Follow-up advice	Reasons for advice
Leave the skin alone for the next 12 hours – it is not even necessary to cleanse it that night	The skin has had an hour-long treatment to deep cleanse and stimulate it, so it is best to allow time for the skin to relax and the salon products to work
Do not apply make-up for 12 hours, if possible	Make-up could clog the skin **pores** and make the skin dirty again before it has had a chance to gain the full benefits of the treatment
Avoid touching the skin	Touching the skin will make it dirty and undo the good work of the facial
Have a monthly facial, if possible	The skin takes about a month to renew its layers, so a regular facial will keep it in great condition
Cleanse, tone and **moisturise**, both morning and evening	This will keep the skin and pores clean and the skin soft
Wear a good moisturiser under make-up and in cold and windy weather	A good moisturiser will protect the skin from getting clogged with make-up and drying out in bad weather
Drink plenty of water and eat a healthy diet with lots of fruit and fresh vegetables	Water will help to **rehydrate** dry skin and a good diet will improve the condition of all skin types
Get plenty of sleep	When we sleep, the skin has a chance to repair itself
Try not to touch or squeeze blackheads and spots	You could make the problem worse and damage the skin
Always protect skin in the sun by using a cream containing a UV-filter (at least SPF 15)	The sun can age and dry out skin

 Top tip

Look ahead to the Anatomy and physiology section in this book and refresh your memory on tips for healthy skin that you can pass on to your client.

Contra-actions

It is also helpful to give the client information on possible **contra-actions**. These are unwanted reactions that could occur, during or after a facial skin care treatment. If these happen during the treatment, the treatment may need to be stopped mid-way through and steps taken to prevent it happening again in the future. If there are no problems during the treatment, you nevertheless need to make the client aware of possible contra-actions in case she experiences them after leaving the salon.

Possible contra-actions to a facial skin care treatment

? Memory jogger

1 Give six points of follow-up advice and the reasons for them.
2 List three possible contra-indications that the client should be aware of before she leaves the salon.

Getting ready for assessment

Evidence requirements

You will be observed by your assessor on at least three occasions, each involving a different client.

What you must cover during your practical assessments

Ranges

In your candidate log book you will have a list of ranges that you must cover during your assessment. These ranges cover:

1 consultation techniques

2 skin types

3 client preparation

4 facial products

5 advice.

It is good practice to cover as many ranges as possible during each assessment. This will prevent you having to take too many additional assessments because there are many ranges that you have not managed to cover.

Performance criteria

What you must demonstrate during a practical observation by your tutor:

- preparation for facials
- a skin analysis
- good communication skills
- basic facial skin care treatment using:
  - cleansers, toners, moisturisers and eye make-up remover
  - tools, equipment and consumables
  - skin care products
  - eye products
- checking the client is happy with the facial skin care treatment
- giving aftercare advice to the client
- leaving the work area in a suitable condition.

Throughout your observations you will also need to make sure that you pay attention to health, safety and hygiene throughout, as well as presenting yourself well, so read through Unit G20 Make sure your own actions reduce risks to health and safety before any practical assessment just to refresh your memory.

Carrying out a practical treatment using unhygienic tools, or without carrying out a risk assessment of your work area to avoid accidents happening, will mean that you are not safe to do a treatment and therefore could mean that you do not pass your assessment.

What you must know

In order to pass this unit, you will need to gather evidence during the teaching and learning of this unit before your assessor observes your practical performance. You will gather this during class work and further study and will probably file it in a portfolio of evidence. This evidence will also be signed off in your candidate log book which you will be given by your assessor. This will be an official record to show that you have covered what you need to.

 Salon life

The senior therapist asked Maz to carry out the cleansing routine on a new client. During the questioning, Maz worked out that the client was 40 years old, but when Maz removed all of the make-up she was quite shocked to see that the client's skin was very yellow and thick and the lines on the face were so much deeper than other mature clients she had treated that actually the client looked more like 60.

While Maz was doing the cleansing routine the client looked up at Maz and complimented her on her complexion, she then asked her where she had got her tan. Maz told her that she sits out in her garden at weekends in the summer and visits the local tanning salon in the winter.

The client then gave Maz a lecture on the dangers of sunbathing and sunbeds and told her that if she continued her skin would look like hers. Maz was shocked!

Find out about the effects of the sun and sunbeds on the skin.

How can Maz learn from her client?

UNIT B3

Assist with day make-up

Make-up can be considered an art form as it allows you to combine imagination and creative thinking to create all kinds of looks using different colour combinations, techniques and styles. There are no set rules other than that you should enhance the client's natural features and give her a look that gives her confidence in her appearance.

In this unit you will learn about safe and hygienic methods of application, carrying out client consultations, make-up application and giving aftercare advice. You will develop practical skills to assist in make-up application while learning about the wide range of make-up products and the use of tools such as brushes, applicators and mixing palettes.

In this unit you will learn how to:

- Maintain safe and effective methods of working when providing day make-up
- Consult and prepare for make-up
- Apply day make-up
- Provide aftercare advice

128

Here are some key terms you will meet in this unit:

Consultation –
a discussion, talk

Lanolin –
a natural oil that comes
from sheep's wool

Anti-bacterial –
something that cuts down
the spread of germs and
infections

Semi-reclining –
lying down but not
completely flat

Allergens –
things that can cause
unwanted allergic
reactions

Psoriasis –
a skin condition consisting
of itchy, dry red patches

Erythema –
abnormal redness
of the skin

Acetone –
a flammable substance
used in nail polish

Dry skin –
skin that is lacking in oil
and may flake and
chap easily

Stipple –
pressing and rolling
action

Dermatitis –
inflammation of
the skin

Combination skin –
skin that is usually made up
of normal and dry skin on the
cheeks and oily skin on the
nose and forehead

Normal skin –
skin that is smooth
with no blemishes

Oily skin –
skin that is shiny with
quite large pores

T-zone –
the nose, chin and forehead,
which can be oily

129

Maintain safe and effective methods of working when providing day make-up (1)

Make-up is no different to any other treatment in a salon. Safety, hygiene and preparation are just as important as they would be for facials or any other treatment.

When you are applying your make-up on yourself at home, it is unlikely that you would think about whether you have used techniques and products that are safe and hygienic. However, when applying make-up on a client, the habits and methods you use at home would probably not be acceptable in the salon.

The work area

Whether you are carrying out your make-up application on a couch or make-up chair, your tutor/assessor will guide you in how to set up your work area and the preparation of the correct products, tools and equipment necessary in the first instance. However, there are essential things that will be required in order to carry out the make-up treatment effectively and these products, tools and equipment are covered on pages 134–135.

The most important requirements are that your set-up is:

- organised – nothing forgotten, all equipment and tools on a trolley, set up in the order of when it will be used
- easy to reach – you will not have to overstretch to reach it or walk across the room
- hygienic – everything is cleaned, disinfected and sterilised, and your couch or chair has a protective cover.

It is very important to be organised with everything to hand as it can be very off-putting to the client if the therapist keeps leaving her to go and fetch something that has been forgotten.

Sterilisation and cleaning of make-up tools and equipment

Where possible you should use disposable applicators for applying make-up as this is the most hygienic method. Make-up brushes should be washed in warm soapy water and left to dry naturally before placing in an ultraviolet cabinet (see Unit G20, pages 20–21 for more details on sterilisation and cleaning methods).

Top tip

It is very easy to spread germs from one client to another by using dirty brushes and towels, putting fingers in pots or setting up on a dirty work surface. This is why sterilisation and hygiene procedures are so important.

Ultraviolet cabinet

All make-up products should be removed from their containers using a disposable spatula or orange stick and placed on a clean make-up palette.

After use the make-up palette should be cleaned with warm soapy water and then wiped over with disinfectant solution.

Lip and eye pencils should be sharpened before use on each client as this means that they have a fresh and sterile surface.

Make-up sponges should be thrown away after use as it is very difficult to clean them thoroughly. If they are reused they should be washed with warm soapy water and left to dry naturally before placing in an ultraviolet cabinet.

✓ Top tip

Don't blow on make-up brushes to remove loose make-up powder before use, as this will make them unhygienic. Instead, shake the loose powder off on to a clean tissue.

» Get up and go!

Make a poster with pictures of your make-up tools and equipment showing how you need to clean, disinfect or sterilise them.

? Memory jogger

1 How do you protect your couch or make-up chair?
2 Why should lip and eye pencils be sharpened before use on each client?
3 What is the best way to clean make-up brushes?
4 How should you remove products from their containers?

131

Maintain safe and effective methods of working when providing day make-up (2)

Maintaining hygiene throughout

It is important to remember that it is not enough to simply follow good hygiene and preparation procedures before you start the treatment. You must ensure that the tools, equipment and yourself remain hygienic throughout the treatment too. (See Unit G20, pages 20–21 for more information on sterilisation and preventing cross-infection.)

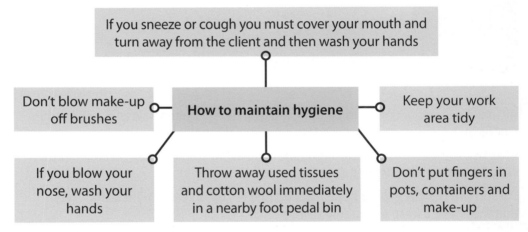

Good hygiene practices

Leaving the work area clean and tidy

If you don't leave your work area clean and tidy it will not be in a fit condition to be used by the next therapist who wishes to carry out another treatment. It goes without saying that a client should not be brought into an untidy and dirty room as this will create a bad impression and could lose the salon customers.

If you have used up equipment and not replaced it, or left the room untidy, the next therapist to use the room will look disorganised and the client may lose confidence in her even though it is not her fault.

Even after you have finished the treatment and your client has left it, hygiene and safety are still important. It is essential that you clear away all of your tools and equipment and that you leave your work area clean and tidy. This includes:

- wiping over trolleys, couches, bins and stools with disinfectant
- washing your brushes and palette
- putting bedding in to be laundered.

Posture and positioning while working

It is important that both you and your client are comfortable throughout the treatment.

All equipment and tools should be within easy reach so that you don't have to overstretch to reach them. The couch or chair should be at the correct height so that you don't have to reach too far up or down.

Your client should be placed in a comfortable position on the couch or chair. She should be able to remain relaxed during the treatment without having to twist or move so that you can reach her.

Celebrity and model make-up artists often apply their make-up using a special chair, called a director's chair. They need to be able to apply perfect make-up in an upright position.

Environmental conditions

Lighting

If the lighting is wrong, the effect of the make-up can be lost. If possible, apply make-up in the same light that the finished result is going to be shown.

For general day make-up, the best form of lighting is daylight. This allows the true colours to show and does not alter the natural colour that is applied. If daylight is not possible, the closest match is natural light bulbs arranged in an arch in front of the client. Professional make-up artists use this light to work in. The client should be positioned in front of the lighting arrangement so that no shadows are cast on her face that could affect the even application of the make-up.

Heating and ventilation

The make-up area should be warm enough so that the client is comfortable and the air conditioning should not make the environment feel stuffy. Clients don't need to undress to have make-up done so it is not necessary to have a very warm area as you would need to for facials.

Get up and go!

Look at your make-up in different lights and see how the colours and effects change. Find out how make-up colours change in:

- daylight
- fluorescent light
- spotlight
- electric light bulbs.

Consult and prepare for make-up (1)

Before starting a make-up treatment, essential preparation is needed to make sure that you know what the client requires, are well prepared and have all the necessary equipment and products. Your equipment and work area must be clean, tidy and hygienic. The basic steps for getting ready for the client's make-up treatment are as follows:

1 Place all equipment and tools on a trolley that is easy to reach; it sometimes helps to lay them out in the order that you will use them so that this also helps to remind you of each step.

2 Set up your couch or chair with protective bedding.

3 Wash your hands.

4 Protect the client's clothing with a make-up cape or draped towel.

5 Protect the client's hair by placing a headband or sterile hair clip around the hairline.

6 Remove any large items of jewellery such as necklaces and earrings that you could accidentally catch.

7 Carry out a **consultation**.

8 If your client wears contact lenses, ask her if she would like to remove them.

9 Position the client in a **semi-reclining** position.

However, the first step before collecting your client is to set up your work area with all the materials that you will need. These are:

- brushes – a range of make-up brushes that you will need
- basics – the disposal products, laundry and workspace requirements
- products – all the creams and lotions needed for the make-up treatment.

Brushes

A good set of brushes is very important, without these you will not be able to complete a professional make-up. Each stage of the make-up needs a different brush.

Face powder brush | Lip liner brush | Contour brush | Eyeliner brush | Mascara wand | Angled eyeshadow brush | Fluff brush | Sponge applicator | Eyebrow brush | Blusher brush

Top tip ✓

You will need to wash your hands again before you start the make-up treatment on the client.

Item	Purpose
Face powder brush	The largest brush used to apply or blend face powder
Blusher brush	Used to apply blusher to the cheek area
Contour brush	Used for shading and highlighting the cheeks and face when you do corrective make-up
Eyebrow brush	A brush one side for brushing brows into shape and a comb the other side for separating lashes
Sponge applicator	Used for applying colour to the eyelids
Mascara wand	Used to apply mascara to the eyelashes
Angled eyeshadow brush	To apply colour or blend colour on the edges or sockets of the eyes
Fluff brush	Completes the blending as it is very soft and gets rid of any unblended edges
Eyeliner brush	To apply eyeliner or for blending eye pencil
Lip liner brush	To apply lipstick smoothly and perfectly

Basics

Item	Purpose
Cotton buds	For correcting any mistakes or make-up smudges
Eye pads (cotton wool circles or squares)	These rest on the eye while using a magnifying mirror for skin analysis
Cotton wool half moons	Cut from damp cotton wool pads, these are placed under the bottom lashes to protect the skin under the eyes from the make-up that is being cleansed off
Damp cotton wool squares	Used to cleanse the face
Tissues	Used for blotting excess toner, moisturiser and the first coat of lipstick
Dry cotton wool	Used to cover the tip of an orange stick which is then used to help remove make-up
Couch roll	Used to protect the client's clothing
Sponge wedges	Made of latex sponge and used to apply foundation to the skin
Make-up cape	Usually a velcro-fastened plastic cape that goes around the client's neck to protect her upper clothes from make-up spills
Headband or turban	To protect the client's hair from the products and to prevent her hair getting in the way of the treatment
Dishes	Small plastic or metal dishes are needed to hold cotton wool, tissues and the client's jewellery
Waste bin	A pedal bin with a lid is best for hygiene purposes, as you can open it without touching it with your hands
Spatula	A wide wooden stick that is used to scoop out cream or lotions from pots. Fingers should never be used as this is unhygienic and could spread germs
Orange sticks	Coat the ends with cotton wool as this softens the tips for safety when cleaning around the eyes
Palette	For decanting products on to and for mixing colours
Sharpener	To sharpen lip and eye pencils

Products

You might use any or all of the following make-up products:

- concealer ▪ foundation ▪ powder ▪ blusher ▪ eyeshadow ▪ eyeliner
- eyebrow pencil ▪ mascara ▪ lip liner ▪ lipstick ▪ lip gloss.

Consult and prepare for make-up (2)

Client consultation

Before beginning any make-up treatment, you need to carry out a client **consultation**. This will involve the following.

- Questioning and recording information: this is when you ask the client questions about her skin and make-up routine and, importantly, why she would like to have her make-up done and what her wishes are. Asking for this information from your client will help you to understand what she needs from the make-up treatment and to find out about any colours or techniques that she does not like.

- Visual analysis: this is when you look at her face shape and skin type, as well as skin and hair colouring, to help you decide techniques and make-up types to use to complement the client's features. It is also important to look for any skin conditions and contra-indications.

- Manual analysis: this is when you feel the skin and decide whether it is dry or oily so that you can match the correct make-up to the skin type.

Remember that good communication skills are essential to conducting a professional consultation. Further information on communication methods can be found in Unit G3 Contribute to the development of effective working reationships.

Top tip ✓

If your client is under the age of 16, a parent or guardian must be present throughout the treatment. The parent or guardian must sign the consultation sheet to agree for the make-up treatment to go ahead – this is called giving consent.

Questioning and recording information

It is important to keep a record of a client's treatment, both during your consultation with the client and when you have completed the treatment.

The example of a consultation card on page 137 shows the information that you would typically record for a make-up treatment and why you need to record it.

» Get up and go!

Look through celebrity magazines and choose a celebrity make-up that you like. Try to copy the look on a friend. Then take a photo of your friend and display it next to the magazine picture in your portfolio so that you can see if they look the same.

MAKE-UP CONSULTATION CARD

DATE 10/09/10   CLIENT'S NAME Mia Shaw

ADDRESS Flat 9, 12 Waterstone,   DATE OF BIRTH 24/03/89
Cambridge CB1 1NS

TELEPHONE NUMBER (H)   019924 555218   (W) 019924 213876

CONDITION OF SKIN ON INSPECTION
Mostly smooth and unlined but with dry patches

CONTRA-INDICATIONS/CONDITIONS
No contra-indications

EYE COLOURS AND PRODUCTS USED
Beige base, medium brown to add depth in the socket
Brown mascara
Brown eyeliner

CHEEK COLOURS AND PRODUCTS USED
Tawny blusher

FOUNDATION AND CONCEALER PRODUCTS AND COLOURS USED
Medium beige foundation and medium stick concealer

LIP COLOURS AND PRODUCTS USED
Nude lip liner and clear lip gloss

REASON FOR MAKE-UP   DAY ☑   EVENING ☐   SPECIAL OCCASION ☐

HOMECARE ADVICE
Use a rich moisturising cream to help the dry patches
Cleanse, tone and moisturise twice daily
Use an eye make-up remover

PRODUCT SALES
Miss Gloss clear lip gloss

COMMENTS
Client really liked the natural day make-up and has booked to come
again as she has a birthday at the end of the month

CLIENT SIGNATURE

RECORD OF TREATMENTS
DATE   TREATMENT   THERAPIST
10/09/10   Day make-up   Pippa Lloyd

It is best to have a record of both the client's first name and surname. It is important to record the first name because there could be two clients with the same surname, which could cause confusion and lead to client records becoming mixed up.

Write the client's full address including the postcode.

Always write down a home number and a work or mobile number. One telephone number is not enough – if a client's appointment needs to be cancelled at short notice, you will not be able to contact her if she is at work and you only have her home telephone number.

Record any contra-indications or allergies in this section.

This is where you record the colours and types of make-up that you apply so that if the client wants the same make-up carried out another time you have the details. The client may also want to buy some of the products so it is important that you or someone else can refer to the record card to find out which products were used.

This is where you record any homecare advice that you give to the client.

This is where you record any products that you sell to the client so that if she returns to buy them again when she runs out the salon has details of what they were.

When you have finished the make-up treatment, this is where you record how you think it went and whether you and the client are happy with the results.

Dates, type of make-up and therapist's name should be kept as it may be useful in the future.

A typical consultation card for a make-up treatment

Consult and prepare for make-up (3)

Visual analysis

Once you have completed the paper-based part of the **consultation**, carried out a first visual study and questioned the client about contra-indications, you will need to thoroughly cleanse the client's skin and carry out a basic skin analysis. This includes finding out about:

- skin type
- skin condition
- contra-indications
- allergies.

This should be done in good light so that you are able to see well the skin's condition and texture.

Skin types and conditions

Skin types and characteristics such as colouring and condition vary between people. The type and characteristics depend on:

- age
- ethnic group
- gender.

When carrying out make-up treatments, you will need to consider all of these things as they will influence the colours, products and techniques that you will use on a client.

Age

Young skin is smooth and blemish-free whereas mature skin has lines and wrinkles, making make-up more difficult to apply.

Ethnic group

Different coloured skin means you will have to consider the colours that you use to complement it. For example, it would be unsuitable to apply a dark foundation colour to a light Caucasian skin.

- Caucasian skin is white and comes mostly from European origins.
- Oriental skin has a yellowish tone and is oily.
- Asian skin has a medium to dark tone with yellow base colour.
- African-Caribbean skin is dark and ranges in colour to almost black.

Gender

Female skin tends to be more sensitive and thinner than male skin, so more care will need to be taken when applying make-up.

Recognising skin types

Normal skin is rarely found in adults. It is usually found in children and young people. It:

- is smooth and clear with no blemishes
- is soft to touch
- has very tiny pores that are difficult to see.

This type of skin needs lots of gentle care to keep it normal.

Oily skin is caused when too much oil is produced in the skin. While we need oil to keep the skin smooth, when the skin produces too much it causes problems. Oily skin:

- has a shiny complexion with blackheads and blemishes
- has pores that are quite large
- means that the skin can be quite thick.

An oily skin can start or become worse as a teenager, when puberty hormones are most active.

Dry skin lacks oil because the oil glands in the skin do not produce enough. It:

- feels tight
- may flake and chap easily after washing, especially if soap is used
- soaks up creams and lotions easily
- can become lined and wrinkled early (especially around the eyes).

Dry skin must be moisturised well. Poor diet and not drinking enough water can cause dry skin or make it worse.

Combination skin is made up of two skin types. These types vary, but the most common is normal or dry skin on the cheek area, and an oily part on the nose and chin, and across the forehead (known as the **T-zone**). The oily T-zone shows up as a shiny nose, chin and forehead with blackheads.

| Normal skin | Oily skin | Dry skin | The **T-zone** |

Matching make-up to a client's skin type

Make-up comes in many forms: pencil, liquid, powder, creams and lotions. It is best to match these where possible to a client's skin type. For example:

- a client with dry or mature skin should have cream-based make-up
- a client with oily skin should have a water-based foundation.

Consult and prepare for make-up (4)

Contra-indications

A contra-indication is a condition that makes or could make a client unsuitable for treatment. Not all contra-indications will prevent a make-up treatment being carried out. Some will just restrict treatment, in other words you can carry on with the make-up but will have to work around the area or go gently taking more care.

Here are some contra-indications that may restrict treatment and some advice for how to adapt your make-up treatment in line with these contra-indications.

- Healed eczema – this will present as very dry and parched skin and can quite often look very lined. Try to apply a very rich moisturiser before applying any make-up.
- **Psoriasis** – this is scaly flakes of skin, quite often red and inflamed. It is best to completely avoid these areas as the make-up will not go on smoothly and could make the condition worse.
- Redness – use a good concealer and covering foundation to balance the redness and steer away from using bright pinks and red, choosing instead neutrals, browns and greys to balance the redness.
- Bruising – use a good concealer to cover the bruising before applying further make-up. Apply it very gently as the bruise may be tender. If it is a very new bruise, you should work around it completely.

However, you must not treat a client who has contra-indications that could be made worse by treatment or could be spread to others.

The contra-indications that prevent you from carrying out your treatment include:

- blisters around the mouth and nose – this could be a cold sore
- bloodshot and watery eyes – this could be an eye infection
- extreme redness and/or inflamation – this could be a sign of an allergy, sunburn or an injury
- swelling or lumps – this could be bruising or something more serious
- dry, red and flaky skin, which could be eczema or **dermatitis**
- healing scars
- cuts
- skin irritation – it is recommended that you postpone the make-up treatment until the irritation goes as it could be a sign of an allergy.

The details about some of the contra-indications on pages 107–109 will help you to know what to look out for.

Dealing with contra-indications

If you notice anything unusual on your client's skin, you should ask your tutor or supervisor to check it for you before you start the treatment. Remember that you should never name a specific contra-indication when encouraging clients to seek medical advice and that you should make sure you do not cause the client to worry.

Contra-actions

Contra-actions are unwanted reactions that could occur during or after a make-up treatment. If these happen during the treatment, the treatment may need to be stopped mid-way through and steps taken to prevent it happening again in the future.

Allergies

Another very important reason why you may not be able to carry out a make-up treatment on your client is if they have an allergy to a product. As a therapist you need to be aware of this and take steps to keep your client safe and healthy.

Ingredients in cosmetics that could cause an allergic reaction include:

- skin care products – soaps and perfumes
- creams and lotions – **lanolin** (generally used in cheaper creams and lotions)
- lipsticks, face powders and blushers – dyes and colourings
- eyeshadows – powdered crushed glass (used to add shimmer)
- mascara and eyeliner – alcohol and fibres
- toning lotions – alcohol or citrus ingredients
- nail polish and removers – **acetone** and alcohol.

It is very difficult to pinpoint which product caused a reaction as you may have used several, but there are medical tests that can be done to find out the cause of the problem.

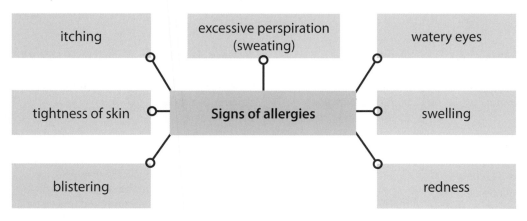

Signs of allergies: itching, excessive perspiration (sweating), watery eyes, tightness of skin, swelling, blistering, redness

 Top tips

- You must always check for allergies before you apply any make-up because many cosmetic products contain **allergens**.

- If, after checking for allergies thoroughly beforehand, a client still reacts badly to a product by showing one of the signs, you will need to remove the product immediately and tell your supervisor, who will decide on the next steps that need to be taken. This will probably be to bathe the area with cool water and advise the client to see her GP.

Consult and prepare for make-up (5)

Preparing the skin

Before you can successfully apply any type of make-up, the skin must be very clean. Application of make-up on skin that has not been thoroughly cleansed and prepared could mean that the make-up will not last as long, will look uneven and will block the pores.

There are four steps to cleansing the skin thoroughly:

1 eye make-up removal **2** cleansing **3** toning **4** moisturising.

Eye make-up remover is a mild cleaning product that dissolves eye make-up so that it can be wiped off. The cleanser will remove old make-up, dirt, dead skin cells and oil from the skin – these also come in special **anti-bacterial** formulations for teenage or oily skin. The toner removes the cleanser, dissolves oil, cools and refreshes the skin while tightening it and closing pores. Finally, application of a moisturiser softens and protects the skin's surface while rehydrating it and providing a smooth base for make-up. You can find more information on all these products in Unit B2 Assist with facial skin care treatments.

Cleansing, toning and moisturising routine

This flow chart illustrates the steps that you should take in order to cleanse, tone and moisturise your client's face in preparation for her make-up treatment.

Start

Cleanse eyes
Place a half moon under the eye to stop the make-up staining the skin. Apply eye make-up remover to the lid using gentle circular movements. Stroke downwards to remove the make-up with a clean damp piece of cotton wool. Repeat until all the eye make-up is removed

Cleanse lips
Apply cleanser to the lips in small circles, using your little finger. Support one side of the mouth and sweep across with a clean piece of cotton wool from this side to the other and back again

Remove cleanser
With damp cotton wool squares

Second cleanse
Follow the routine illustrated on page 143 once more

Skin analysis
Look carefully at the skin to find out about the skin type, condition and texture

Remove cleanser
With damp cotton wool squares using the same routine

First facial cleanse
Follow the routine illustrated on page 143

Apply toner
Put onto damp cotton wool and follow the cleansing routine to apply it

Blot toner
Using a split tissue, place it on the skin to soak up the excess toner

Repeat toning and blotting

Apply moisturiser
Apply using cleansing routine strokes

Wait for five minutes
Leave the skin to settle for five minutes and to give the moisturiser time to sink in. This is a good time to chat with your client about make-up colours

Finish

This diagram illustrates in detail the cleansing routine that you should follow.

Decant enough cleanser onto your hand to complete the first cleanse, spread it out between your hands and start the cleansing routine below.

1 Four stroking effleurage on the neck

2 Four stroking effleurage on the right cheek

3 Four stroking effleurage on the chin

4 Four stroking effleurage on the left cheek

5 Circles around the chin

6 Petrissage circles around the mouth and nose

7 Four stroking effleurage on the bridge of the nose

8 Four stroking effleurage on the forehead

9 Four eye circles (go in the direction of the eyebrow)

10 Finish with pressure on the temples before lifting hands off

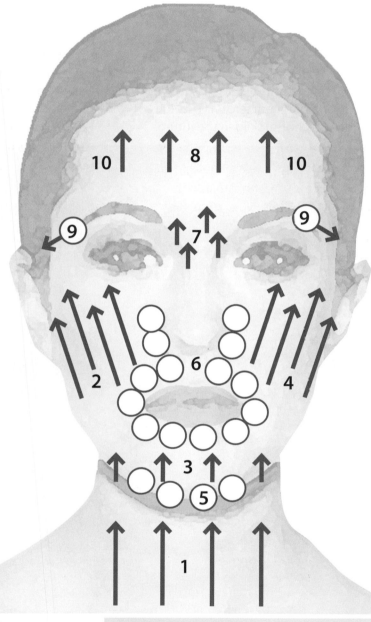

Cleansing routine

Move upwards, keeping in contact with the skin – do not lift your hands off

>> **Get up and go!**

Find out about where the words effleurage and petrissage come from.

? **Memory jogger**

1 What would happen if you applied make-up on uncleansed skin?

2 Give two disorders that may restrict a make-up treatment.

3 What is the difference between a contra-indication and a contra-action?

4 In what order should you carry out a make-up treatment?

   A Cleanse, skin analysis, tone, moisturise, make-up

   B Cleanse, tone, moisturise, make-up, skin analysis

   C Skin analysis, cleanse, tone, make-up, moisturise

   D Skin analysis, cleanse, make-up, moisturise, tone

For step-by-step photos of how to cleanse, tone and moisturise a client's face, please turn to pages 116–121 in Unit B2 Assist with facial skin care treatments.

Apply day make-up (1)

Although make-up may be used for a variety of effects such as theatre, television and photography, the techniques covered in this section are the first steps to developing skills as a make-up artist.

As with most things in life, for some people, make-up application comes naturally, whereas for others it can take a long time to perfect. At this stage, what is most important is to take care to not rush the application, and to think carefully about how to enhance the client's features and natural appearance. The steps and information outlined here will provide you with a solid base for developing more advanced technical skills in the future.

You need to think carefully about how to enhance features and create a natural appearance

Sequence of make-up application

To some extent, there are no set rules for the order in which you should apply make-up. It really depends on the products that are being used and the effect that is required. However, a common-sense approach to make-up application is important. The routine shown below would be a sensible way to go about it.

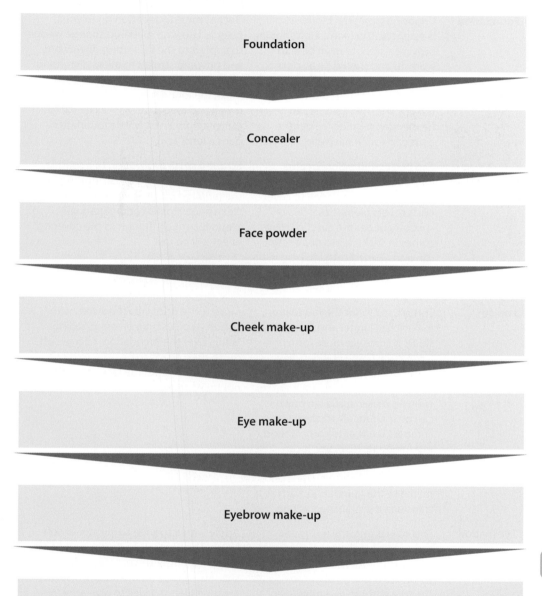

Foundation

Concealer

Face powder

Cheek make-up

Eye make-up

Eyebrow make-up

Lip make-up

A make-up routine

Some people prefer to apply eye make-up before cheek make-up and this is acceptable. However, if cream eye make-up or cream cheek make-up is used, this should be applied before face powder and not afterwards as in the routine above.

 Top tip

Never rush the first stages of foundation, concealer and powder application. It is these stages that prepare the skin for the colour – think of it as preparing your painting canvass.

145

Apply day make-up (2)

Make-up products and application

Product	The basics	Application
Foundation	Choosing the correct foundation is essential. The foundation should provide a smooth even base to work on and should be as close to the natural skin tone as possible. You should test the colour on the jaw line. Two colours can be blended together to get the correct colour if necessary.	Decant some foundation on to your palette. Use your make-up sponge wedge to apply it to the face using downward and outward strokes to avoid disturbing the tiny hairs on the face which could make the foundation go blotchy. Blend it well and fade it out at the jawline to prevent hard lines. A little foundation goes a long way.
Concealer	Can be applied before or after foundation depending on the type and how much you need to cover up. It covers blemishes, scars or shadows under the eye. Concealer comes in sticks, tubes or jars and can also be medicated to help with spots. It has a similar texture to foundation but is thicker.	Scrape a small amount on to a spatula, apply to skin using a brush, dotting in the required place. Then **stipple** using clean fingertips, blending gradually. Don't blend too much though as the covering effect will be lost.
Powder	This is used to set the foundation, make it last longer and to cut down shine. It comes in loose form or in a compact. Some powders have glitter or pearlised ingredients added to them, which are great for evening make-up. Loose powder can be used for all occasions, but compact is easier to carry around in a handbag. However, it can be unhygienic so should not be used by lots of people. Use a good match to the foundation, such as a translucent or transparent one.	Apply loose or compact powder with cotton wool, using a pressing/rolling action over the foundation. A large soft brush then needs to be used to brush off extra powder from the face so that it does not look too thick.
Eyeshadow	This comes in many forms and there are a whole range of colours and textures for use on the eyes. Eyeshadow brings colour to the face and can minimise less attractive facial features. Eye make-up can be used to correct features such as deep-set eyes. Effects can be soft or dramatic depending on the client's wishes or occasion, and it is not necessary to use the same colour as the eyes as they contain many different flecks of colour naturally.	Apply with a sponge applicator or soft brush. The lightest shade, the highlighter, is applied under the brow and the darker shadow colours on the lid. Eyeshadow must be blended well to give a soft appearance and professional finish.

Product	The basics	Application
Highlighter	This is usually powder-based and is a light colour such as white, beige or cream. It is used to highlight features.	Apply this to the arch of the eye with an eyeshadow applicator to open up the eyes. Also apply it to the cheeks using a blusher brush – it should be placed just above your blusher.
Eyeliner	Eyeliners go in and out of fashion regularly and are used to draw attention to the eyes. Eyeliner can be used to open, lengthen or add depth to the eyes depending on the type of application and colour. There are many types – liquid, cake, pencil or pen applicator.	Apply in a fine line as close to the roots of the lashes as possible. It can be applied to both the top and bottom lashes or either. To prevent hard lines, blend into eyeshadow by applying eyeshadow softly over the top. Use a damp cotton wool bud to clean up any smudges or mistakes.
Mascara	This makes the lashes look fuller and longer and comes in many colours and types; for example, some have fibres, some are waterproof. Some mascara can cause problems for clients with sensitive eyes or contact lens wearers, so always check for contra-indications and allergies before using.	Apply first downwards over the upper lashes, then ask client to look up slightly and stroke them upwards to coat underneath. Then coat the lower lashes. Keep a clean mascara comb so that you can separate any lashes that join together. Apply mascara in several thin coats rather than one thick coat and allow to dry between coats.
Blusher	This is used to give soft colour to the cheeks, create better shape and correct face shapes.	Apply powder blusher after the powder and cream blushers before powder. Apply with a brush to the cheek area, building up the colour slowly until you are happy with the result. Heavily applied blusher looks unnatural.
Lip liner	This is used to give a smooth outline to the lips and to correct the shape. Use a colour close to the natural lip colour if using a pale lipstick or clear lip gloss or, if using a brighter lipstick, use a liner the same colour.	Rest your little finger on the client's chin for support and gently outline the lips with the pencil. Do not ask the client to stretch her lips because when they relax and go back to normal the liner will be uneven and too dark.
Lipstick	This is the final touch to a make-up and brings the whole effect together. It adds colour and texture to the face as well as gloss and shine to the lips. Lipstick comes in many colours and textures, ranging from cream to pearlised and matt to glossy.	Scrape a little off of the stick with a spatula and apply using a lip brush. Coat the outer part of the lips first and then fill in the centre. Blot with a tissue and then apply a second coat – this will give a better coverage and make the lipstick last longer.
Lip gloss	If applied to bare lips it gives a beautiful sheen or if used on top of lipstick it enhances the lipstick. It comes in many forms and colours.	Apply evenly with a lip brush, taking care not to overload the lips.

Apply day make-up (3)

Consequences of applying unsuitable make-up products

If make-up is applied incorrectly, the skin could suffer. Heavy-handed application of products could bruise the skin and it could also become sore and irritated. If a very sharp eye pencil was used around the eye, this could scratch the delicate skin around the eyes.

As well as poor application techniques, the wrong sort of make-up would be unsuitable. Deeply moisturising products on an oily skin would mean that the make-up would not last as it would come off easily. On the other hand, water-based products on dry flaky skin could make the make-up look patchy and uneven. Waterproof mascara that is difficult to remove or mascara with fibres in it could affect sensitive eyes. Using the wrong colours for skin type and characteristics will result in an unattractive make-up finish that is not right for the client.

Contra-actions

These are unwanted reactions to the make-up treatment. Certain products or techniques can cause problems, such as:

- redness
- rash
- soreness.

If your client shows any sign of these after you have applied a make-up product, you must remove it straight away and bathe the skin with cool water. The contra-action should calm down fairly quickly.

Other contra-actions that could happen are excessive perspiration, otherwise known as sweating, watery eyes and **erythema** (extreme redness).

How to treat contra-actions

Sweating: lower the temperature of the room, open a window, give the client a cool drink and stop the treatment until the sweating stops.

Watery eyes: give the client a tissue to dab at her eyes and wait until the watering stops before continuing with the eye make-up.

Erythema: this could be a sign of an allergy so stop using the make-up, remove it and bathe the skin with cool water.

Top tips

- Always work with clean, sterilised equipment to prevent germs spreading.
- Work with care around the eyes as they are very delicate.

? Memory jogger

1 Give three examples of contra-actions.
2 Give three examples of contra-indications to make-up treatment.
3 Give three occasions when a client may want a make-up done.
4 Why should make-up be applied in a certain order?

Step-by-step make-up

1 Prepare the client for her make-up treatment.

2 Apply foundation with a latex sponge wedge downwards and outwards.

3 Apply concealer with a small brush and **stipple** it with a clean finger to blend.

4 Set foundation and concealer by applying powder in a pressing and rolling action with a ball of cotton wool and dust the excess with a large soft powder brush.

Apply day make-up (4)

Step-by-step make-up

5   Apply blusher sparingly to prevent colour build up and a hard appearance.

6   Use a sponge applicator to apply the highlighter under the brow bone.

7   Add darker colour/s to the lid and blend afterwards with a soft eye brush.

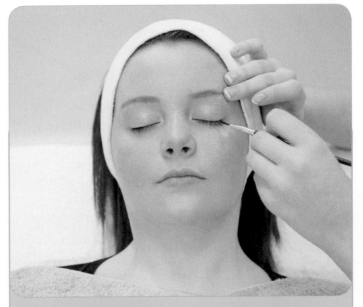

8   Apply eyeliner in a fine line as close to the lashes as possible. Blend with the eyeshadow to soften hard lines if desired. Then apply an eye pencil or shadow under the lashes to balance the eyes.

9 Apply mascara to the lashes using even, light strokes and comb through with a lash comb to separate the hairs.

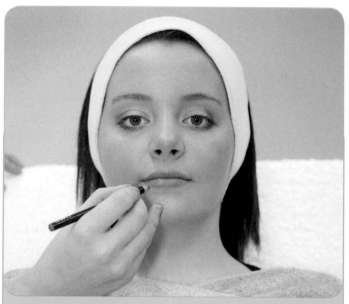

10 Balance your hand on the chin and gently apply the lip liner on the outside of the lips.

11 Complete the look by applying lipstick and lip gloss with a clean brush.

12 Show the client the mirror so that she can see the finished result.

Provide aftercare advice

It is important to remember that a treatment is not complete unless you have given your client some good advice for her to follow at home.

 Salon life

Emma was so pleased she had completed her first make-up on a client without the senior therapist helping her. She applied the make-up perfectly and her special sparkly mascara from her own make-up bag really set off the whole look. Emma's client went home thrilled with her make-up knowing that she would look great with her little black dress on for the party tonight.

However, as Emma's client was getting dressed her eyes and the skin around them started to itch. When she looked in the mirror her eyes had started to swell and were bloodshot. She looked dreadful and her flatmate gasped in horror. She rushed to the bathroom and rubbed off all her eye make-up, but the swelling did not go down – it just got worse.

Did Emma do anything wrong?

What should Emma's client do?

Had Emma's client been given enough information about how to deal with contra-actions?

Checking client satisfaction

A satisfied client will hopefully be a returning client, whether for make-up or something else, so it is important that you not only use good communication skills throughout the treatment but that you check that she is satisfied with what you have done.

During the application it is a good idea to check:

- that she is comfortable and warm
- that she is happy with the application so far – show her the progress in the mirror.

At the end of the treatment:

- show her the finished result in the mirror
- ask her if she is happy or if there is anything she would like slightly changed
- show her and explain the products that you used and where and how you used them
- offer to write the products down for her so that if she decides she would like to buy them she knows which ones to buy.

Homecare advice

Remember to give the following follow-up advice.

- Advise her not to touch her face too much as it will rub off the make-up.
- Advise her to make her make-up last longer by re-applying some powder and lipstick throughout the day.
- Advise her to remove her make-up very thoroughly before going to bed.
- Tell your client that if she has any contra-actions when she gets home or up to a couple of days afterwards, such as itchiness, irritation, redness or flaking, it may be that her skin has reacted to one of the make-up products. She will need to inform the salon and if the problem gets worse she must visit her GP.

Make-up removal techniques

Advise your client to gently use eye make-up remover, massaging it around the eye in circular movements and then using a cotton wool ball to remove the make-up and the eye make-up remover, taking care not to drag the eyes down.

For the face make-up, advise her on cleansing, toning and moisturising to ensure that all traces of make-up are removed and not left to block the pores.

Recording the treatment

All the techniques and colours used should be written on the client consultation card so that if the client returns for the same treatment you have a reference of the make-up used. She may also visit to buy some of the make-up products and if you have not written these down it is likely that you will have forgotten what you used.

Get ahead

Design a make-up consultation card that can be given to a client at the end of her treatment. It should record the products used and how to use them.

Get up and go!

Design your own make-up demonstration chart, with actual make-up colour smears, showing all of the colours that complement each other and that would blend well.

? Memory jogger

1 List three homecare pieces of advice that you could give to your client.
2 How can you check that the client is satisfied with the make-up treatment?
3 Describe how to remove eye make-up.

Getting ready for assessment

Evidence requirements

You will be observed by your assessor on at least three occasions, each involving a different client.

What you must cover during your practical assessments

Ranges

In your candidate log book you will have a list of ranges that you must cover during your assessment. These ranges cover:

1 **consultation** techniques
2 skin types
3 client preparation
4 make-up products
5 advice.

It is good practice to cover as many ranges as possible during each assessment. This will prevent you having to take too many additional assessments because there are many ranges that you have not managed to cover.

Performance criteria

What you must demonstrate during a practical observation by your tutor:

- preparation for make-up
- a skin analysis
- good communication skills
- basic make-up application using:
  - foundation
  - concealers
  - powder
  - eye products
  - cheek products
  - lip products.
- checking the client is happy with the make-up treatment and finished effect
- giving aftercare advice to the client
- leaving the work area in a suitable condition.

Throughout your observations you will also need to make sure that you pay attention to health, safety and hygiene throughout, as well as presenting yourself well, so read through Unit G20 Make sure your own actions reduce risks to health and safety before any practical assessment just to refresh your memory.

Top tips

- Make sure you are confident and have organised your work area, tools and equipment well.
- Prepare a checklist so that it is easy to check that you have everything to hand.
- Concentrate, don't let friends distract you.

Carrying out a practical treatment using unhygienic tools, or without carrying out a risk assessment of your work area to avoid accidents happening, will mean that you are not safe to do a treatment and therefore could mean that you do not pass your assessment.

What you must know

In order to pass this unit, you will need to gather evidence during the teaching and learning of this unit before your assessor observes your practical performance. You will gather this during classwork and further study and will probably file it in a portfolio of evidence. This evidence will also be signed off in your candidate log book which you will be given by your assessor. This will be an official record to show that you have covered what you need to.

 Salon life

Jemima had an assessment today but had forgotten her make-up kit. Luckily she had her own make-up in her school bag so laid this out on her trolley when she was setting up for her client. Her friend Lucy lent Jemima some disposable eyeshadow applicators and lipliner brush, but did not have a disposable mascara brush.

Jemima started to apply a lovely day make-up using her own make-up and making do with the brushes she had in her own bag.

How could Jemima spread germs to her client by using her own make-up and brushes?

What infections could she pass on to her client by using her own make-up and mascara brush?

>> Get up and go!

Cut out examples of make-up on celebrities from your magazines. Label the ones you like and say why, and the ones you don't like and say why.

Discuss with a partner how they could be improved.

UNIT N1

Assist with nail services

Well cared-for hands and nails are a great confidence booster. When a client looks down at her nails after a nail care treatment, she will notice a big improvement, even if she cares for them well herself. A professional nail care treatment is steps ahead of do-it-yourself treatments.

In this unit you will learn how to help with nail treatments and care for the nails on the hands and feet and surrounding skin. You will also learn about preparing for treatments and advising clients on aftercare.

In this unit you will learn how to:

- Maintain safe and effective methods of working when assisting with nail services
- Consult, plan and prepare for nail services with clients
- Carry out nail services
- Provide aftercare advice

Here are some key terms you will meet in this unit:

Cuticle –
hardened skin at the base of the fingernail

Manual labour –
work involving the hands

Scarf nail –
fine wisps of nail that stick out after soaking

Methodical –
careful and organised, paying attention to detail

Nail plate –
the hard, visible part of the fingernail

Verruca –
a wart caused by a virus, commonly found on the feet and very infectious

Stress points –
the parts where the nail is weakest

Athlete's foot –
a fungal infection commonly found on the feet

Abrasive –
a rough and scratchy substance that is used to clean a smooth surface

Manicure station –
a trolley designed especially for carrying out manicures

Bevelling –
a method of filing the nails to reduce splitting

Hangnails –
dry strips of skin at the sides of the nail that can become very sore and inflamed if left untreated or pulled off

Buffing –
polish and make shiny

Matrix –
the root of the nail

Pumice stone –
a special foot care tool designed to remove hard skin

Maintain safe and effective methods of working when assisting with nail services [1]

Nail care treatments involve very close work and close attention to safe working practices is very important. However carefully you look after your nails at home, it is unlikely that you follow the high standards of hygiene expected of salon treatments. Some nail treatments use electrical equipment such as nail drills, files and dust extractors, which means that when you are assisting a therapist you need to be able to recognise safe working methods and follow instructions, even though you probably will not use electrical equipment yourself, as you may help to set them up.

The work area

Manicures

A manicure can be carried out in a variety of ways and some of these are better than others.

Some salons have an area especially set up for manicures, with good lighting and all equipment and products at hand. This is the best practice for manicure treatments.

In other salons a manicure is carried out in the reception area or as an extra part of a treatment. This is not best practice, and can be awkward for both the client and the therapist.

Here are the ways that a manicure can be carried out.

- Across a couch – with the client on one side and you on the other, and the products laid out next to you.

- At a **manicure station** – this is a trolley on wheels designed especially for carrying out manicures. It usually has drawers for storage and sometimes has a magnifying lamp. There should be room for the client to sit one side of the station and for the therapist to sit on the other side.

- The client sits in a couch or chair while the therapist sits on a manicure stool. The manicure stool has a cushioned seat, a swinging arm for resting and supporting the client's hands and arms and drawers underneath for the storage of products.

- The therapist sits to the side of the client while she is having her hair done. This is a very unsatisfactory way of carrying out a manicure. It is difficult for the therapist to carry out the manicure in comfort, which could affect the standard of the manicure.

- The therapist sits to the side of the treatment couch while the client has a facial. Again, this is not the best way to carry out a manicure. Either the client will have to stretch one of her arms across her body, or the therapist will have to swap sides to carry out the treatment on the second hand.

Pedicures

Setting up for a pedicure is more straightforward. The client usually sits on a professional chair that has a supportive back and the therapist sits in front.

Best practice is where the client's feet can rest on a special foot rest for pedicures. If a special foot rest is not available then the client can rest her feet on the therapist's lap, but this is less comfortable for both client and therapist.

Alternatively, well-equipped salons will have an electric-pedicure station, which is a large chair with built in foot bath and back massage facility for the client to enjoy during her pedicure.

As for any treatment, your work area must be organised with everything easy for you to reach. All items must be hygienic, with everything cleaned, disinfected and sterilised. Organise your products and tools in advance, and remember that it is helpful to arrange them in the order in which you will use them.

Top tip

When you set up, make sure that the tools and equipment are positioned so that you don't have to bend over to reach them. If you are right-handed, position the tools and equipment on the left. If you are left-handed, position them on the right. This helps to prevent you from knocking things over.

Get up and go!

Investigate a range of salon suppliers on the Internet to find out the different types of manicure and pedicure tools and equipment available for salons to buy. Print off some pictures of these for your portfolio.

Maintain safe and effective methods of working when assisting with nail services (2)

Sterilisation and cleaning of nail care tools and equipment

Maintaining standards of hygiene during nail treatments is extremely important. It is very easy to cause infection by using dirty tools and equipment. You must at all costs avoid allowing bacteria to enter the growing part of the nail through the **cuticle** or breaks in the skin.

Unit G20 Make sure your own actions reduce risks to health and safety explains in detail the difference between cleaning, disinfection and sterilisation, so refer back to this unit.

When setting up for nail treatments, you must follow these rules.

- All equipment must be cleaned with a detergent and then sterilised. The detergent removes the dirt and debris from their surfaces.
- Tools that need to be sterilised are things like cuticle knives, nippers and hard skin removers.
- All work surfaces must be disinfected using a spray or by wiping over with a disinfectant solution.
- Clean towels must be provided for each client and a biological detergent used so that they don't have to be washed at a very high temperature, which is not environmentally friendly.
- All creams, lotions and sprays used throughout the treatment should be decanted from pump-action bottles so that they are less likely to become contaminated with bacteria. If these are not available, a spatula must be used instead to remove the products from the container, bottle, tub or tube.
- Washing hands reduces the growth of germs and bacteria and also removes dust and dirt. Use a liquid soap in a pump-action bottle and paper towels as this is the most hygienic method. Always dry them thoroughly after washing as wet hands are not clean hands.

The table below shows how cross-infection could occur during a nail treatment.

Stage of the manicure or pedicure	Unhygienic practices that could lead to cross-infection	Potential result
Preparing to treat the client and/or during the whole of the treatment	Completing a treatment on one client and then carrying straight on to the next client without washing your hands, or handling money (money is covered in many germs) and then treating a client without washing your hands, or going to the toilet during the treatment and returning to the client without washing your hands.	Illness and skin infections
Soaking nails in warm soapy water	Using water that has previously been used on another client. The previous client may have had a **verruca**, or there may now be bits of skin floating in the water, either from the soles of the feet or the fingernails, which contain germs and dirt.	Veruccas and other bacterial, and fungal conditions such as **athlete's foot** and ringworm
Pushing back **cuticles**	Using cuticle tools that have not been sterilised and are covered in germs, which are then used on different clients.	Swollen and infected cuticles
Moisturising hands and feet	Using your fingers instead of a disposable spatula to scoop out the cream from the pot, meaning that after a few treatments the cream is full of germs from different clients.	Skin infections

Remember that the results of not being hygienic could be very damaging for both the salon and your career.

Maintaining hygiene throughout

You must remember that tools, equipment and you need to stay clean and hygienic throughout the treatment. The good hygiene and preparation procedures that you followed before starting are not enough, so you will need to make sure that:

- if you sneeze or cough you must cover your mouth and turn away from the client and then go and wash your hands
- if you blow your nose, wash your hands
- you don't put fingers in pots and containers of cream
- if you drop any nail tools or equipment, they must be cleaned and sterilised again
- you keep your work area tidy
- you throw away used tissues and cotton wool immediately in a nearby bin.

Leaving the work area clean and tidy

After you have finished the treatment and your client has left it is essential that you clear away all of your tools and equipment and that you leave your work area clean and tidy. This will include:

- wiping over trolleys, couches, bins and stools with disinfectant
- cleaning your manicure tools and implements
- putting bedding in to be laundered
- tidying the work area for the next treatment or service.

»» Get up and go!

Search the Internet for instructions and pictures showing how to wash your hands correctly. Choose the clearest picture and instructions, print it off and laminate it. Then put it by the sink in your classroom so that you have clear waterproof instructions for everyone to follow.

? Memory jogger

1 List three ways that you could cause cross-infection during your nail treatment.
2 What sort of detergent should be used to wash towels?
3 What are the three methods of reducing germs and bacteria?

161

Maintain safe and effective methods of working when assisting with nail services (3)

Checking that your equipment is in good working order

All equipment should be checked before starting the treatment so that it is safe to use, clean and works properly. You will need to check with your senior therapist or supervisor to make sure that everything is in good working order. Using poorly prepared equipment increases the risk of accidents in the workplace whereas dirty equipment could spread bacteria and cause infections.

Posture and positioning while working

As for any professional treatment, it is important that both you and your client are comfortable throughout the treatment.

During manicures and pedicures the therapist needs to bend over to carry out the service more so than other treatments, so it is especially important that you pay attention to your posture. It is important that you make sure that both you and your client are comfortable and that the height of the nail or pedicure station is easy to reach and does not make you lean over or bend too much. If your back is overstretched from reaching when carrying out the treatment, it will cause you back pain, neck ache and tiredness.

Therefore, once you have decided where you will be carrying out your nail service, you must make sure that:

- you and the client are not too cramped – there should be plenty of room for both of you to move your arms and legs freely
- the client is not positioned too far from you. You must be able to reach her hands and arms without having to lean over or stretch up.

Environmental conditions

Lighting

In order to see the **nail plate**, **cuticles** and polish during a manicure or pedicure, good overhead or natural lighting is essential. When carrying out the treatment, you should always check the following.

- Is the light bright enough?
- Does the light cast shadows?

This may be a particular problem if you are positioned in the corner of a room.

 Get up and go!

Set up for a nail treatment and then test different types of lighting on the area to see how much and how clearly you can see your tools, equipment and the nails of a friend.

Heating and ventilation

During nail treatments clients don't need to undress, but they will still take off their coat. For pedicures they will also either remove their trousers or skirt, or roll them up out of the way, so it is quite easy for them to get cold. Use a towel as a warm covering as well as for protection.

Although basic nail care treatments do not produce a lot of dust and vapour like artificial nail treatments, there is still the possibility that products such as nail varnish removers, acetone and varnishes could produce fumes that could overcome client and therapist. For this reason it is advisable to allow fresh air to circulate and during the winter, when perhaps this is not possible, a suitable method of artificial ventilation needs to be used.

Because of the possibility of fumes you must remember to replace bottle tops immediately after use and use a pedal bin that closes properly for your waste.

 Top tip

Never leave cotton wool that is soaked in nail varnish remover on the work top. It will not only begin to dissolve a plastic nail station, it will also give off unwanted fumes.

 Memory jogger

1 What products could cause fumes during nail treatments?

2 How can you cut down fumes?

3 What is ventilation?

4 Why is it more likely for your back to ache during nail care treatments?

Consult, plan and prepare for nail services with clients (1)

The two keys to any successful nail treatment are good organisation and careful consideration of your client's needs. Clients will come to the salon for nail treatments for different reasons, so it is important for you to find out exactly what your client's wishes are. You will also need to look carefully at the nails and surrounding skin so that you can determine their condition and the nail shape, identify any problems and record details of the nail care routine that she follows at home. All this will help you to plan a treatment suitable for your client.

However, the first step before consulting with your client is to prepare your work area and set it up with all the materials that you will need. These are:

- basics – the disposable products, laundry and workspace requirements
- tech tools – the tools, such as scissors, that you will need
- products – all the creams and lotions needed for the treatment.

All of the basics, tech tools and products that you will need to assist with nail services are listed and explained on pages 165–167. Look back at pages 20–21 of Unit G20 Make sure your own actions reduce risks to health and safety to remind yourself of the correct procedures for cleaning, disinfecting and sterilising tools and work surfaces.

To make sure that you keep the tools and equipment needed for nail services in good working order, make sure that you:

- clean and sterilise them after every client
- only use tools made for professional nail services
- oil the hinges and screws regularly to stop them becoming stiff.

Top tip

It helps to have a checklist of the tech tools, products and nail basics on a record card that you can keep nearby for reference. Cover the list with a plastic cover so that it does not get marked, or have it laminated so that you can wipe it clean.

Get ahead

Design and carry out a survey to find out how often clients have their nails done professionally and the sorts of nail services they have. Discuss the findings with your friends and tutor.

Basics

Item	Purpose
Cotton wool	To remove nail varnish, the cotton wool is rolled into small balls and each ball is soaked with nail varnish remover. A clean piece of cotton wool is used for each nail. Cotton wool is also used to cover the tip of an orange stick, for **cuticle** work, the application of cream and nail cleaning.
Tissues	Tissues are used for various things during a manicure, such as wiping products from the nail. Tissues are normally made up of two very thin layers (two-ply). In a salon, tissues are split (one-ply) as this makes them more economical to use.
Towels	A towel is used to dry the hands and fingers or feet and toes of the client after they have been soaked in water during a manicure or pedicure. Towels are also used to protect a client's clothing if she is not wearing a gown.
Gown	The client may wear a gown to protect her clothing from spills or splashes of a product, or you may place a protective towel over her clothing instead.
Dishes	Small plastic or metal dishes are needed to hold cotton wool and tissues, as well as the client's jewellery. Any jewellery left on during a manicure will get in the way of the treatment and become coated in hand cream.
Waste bin or container	A pedal bin with a lid is best for hygiene purposes, as you can open it without touching it with your hands. However, if you are doing a manicure or pedicure in a corner of a room or an area without a pedal bin, then you can use a waste paper bin lined with a disposable bag. After the treatment, make sure that the bin is emptied, and the bag is sealed and placed in a waste bin with a lid. If a bowl or container other than a bin is used for waste, make sure that you have lined it with couch roll first. This will allow you to scoop the waste up easily after the treatment. Remember to wash and disinfect the bowl afterwards.
Sterilising jar	This should be filled with antiseptic or disinfectant solution, so that small metal tools that have been previously sterilised can be placed in it during the treatment. The solution will help to keep germ levels down, but it will not destroy germs completely. The solution should be changed after every client.
Manicure cushion	These provide extra comfort during the manicure. They allow the client to rest her hands and also give support to the wrist. Cushions are not usually used for pedicures as the foot is supported on a foot stool or pedicure station. Manicure cushions usually have a removable washable cover made from towelling. However, if the cushion does not have a cover, then a protective towel should be placed on top.
Manicure or pedicure bowl	The manicure bowl is a specially shaped gripper bowl, which has a small hole in it for the thumb and a larger hole for the rest of the fingers. It is filled with warm soapy water in which to soak the client's hands during the manicure. It has a removable lid so that it can be cleaned thoroughly inside after each treatment. For the pedicure a shaped foot bowl is sometimes used, or at other times a foot spa or built-in foot bath.

Consult, plan and prepare for nail services with clients (2)

Tech tools

When setting up for a nail service, you need to prepare all the tools you will need.

Item	Purpose
Spatula	A spatula is used for scooping out products hygienically.
Emery board	This is a thin card file with an **abrasive** covering on each side. It is used for filing and shaping the nails. The fine side is used for fingernails and the coarse side for male manicures and toenails, as they tend to be thicker than fingernails. Emery boards come in different sizes and widths, and some have funky designs on them. They should be disposed of after use, for hygiene purposes.
Orange sticks	These are made of orange wood, which is slightly bendy. One end is pointed and the other end is shaped like a hoof. Both ends of the orange stick are coated in cotton wool for hygiene purposes, as the cotton wool can be removed and thrown away after use. The cotton wool also softens the tip, which prevents the **cuticles** and skin becoming sore during treatment. The pointed end is used for cleaning under the free edge of the nail and the hoof end is used for cuticle work.
Rubber hoof stick	In addition to the orange stick, this tool can also be used to push back the **cuticles** safely. At the end of the wooden stick is a hoof-shaped rubber piece. However, once it has been sterilised a few times, the rubber tends to fall apart, so the hoof stick needs to be replaced regularly.
Nail brush	This can be used during the nail soaking to gently rub away staining around the fingers or toes or on the nails. It is also used to take off cuticle remover. However, it is not a very hygienic tool as it is extremely difficult to sterilise completely and can harbour germs between the bristles.
Nail buffer	This is made of chamois leather and is used with a buffing paste to shine the **nail plate**. The action of the **buffing** also improves the blood flow to the nails, which encourages nail growth.
Nail scissors	These are curved scissors that can be used to cut long nails before filing if it would take too long to use an emery board.
Cuticle knife	This blunt, straight-edged tool is used to gently free any cuticle that has stuck to the nail plate. This is done by applying light pressure and making small circular movements at the base of the nail. When using this tool, you should be careful not to use a digging and pushing-back action, as this will only damage the **matrix** and make the cuticles sore. You should know about the instrument, but you will not be using it at Level 1.
Cuticle nippers	These cutting tools do not cut the main part of the cuticle, as the name suggests. Instead, they are used gently to cut away extra skin that has grown down the nail from dry, uncared-for cuticles. They are used only after the cuticle has been softened and loosened with cuticle remover and a hoof stick or cuticle knife. You should know about the instrument, but you will not be using it at Level 1.

Products

When setting up for a nail service, you need to make sure you have all the products you will need.

Product	Purpose
Nail varnish	This is used to colour or give shine to the nails at the end of the nail care treatment. They come in many colours, effects and types.
Nail varnish remover	This dissolves nail varnish so that it can be wiped off the **nail plate** easily with a piece of cotton wool. Nail varnish remover has a drying effect on the nail so it usually contains a small amount of oil to moisturise it.
Cuticle cream	This is a thick moisturising cream that is used to soften and nourish the **cuticle** so that the cuticle can be pushed back more easily during a nail care treatment without the skin splitting or pulling.
Cuticle remover	This is a milky-coloured liquid that contains an active ingredient to dissolve skin cells. It is used to loosen any **cuticle** that sticks to and grows along the nail plate. It also acts as a nail shampoo because it contains an active ingredient to bleach out stains. The senior therapist will demonstrate and carry out this part of the nail treatment.
Buffing paste	**Buffing** paste contains an **abrasive** ingredient that is used to smooth out fine ridges on the surface of the nail. It also helps to remove surface stains on the nail plate. Buffing paste leaves the nails with a shiny surface and can be used instead of nail varnish.
Moisturiser or massage cream	This is a rich cream that is massaged into the hands and arms or feet and lower legs at the end of the manicure or pedicure and before the nail varnish is applied.
Nail varnish dryer	A nail varnish dryer does not dry the nails completely, but it helps the varnish to harden more quickly. It comes in the form of a spray or paint-on-product (similar to clear nail varnish) and can be oil- or alcohol-based.

>> **Get up and go!**

How many nail basics, lotions and creams, and tech tools can you remember? In pairs, look at each list for one minute. Then test each other's memory.

? **Memory jogger**

1 How should you cut a nail to prevent damage to the layers?
2 Name two tools that you will not use for Level 1.
3 The skin around the nails is removed with:
   A Cuticle remover
   B Cuticle massage cream
   C Acetone
   D Buffing paste
4 Give two uses of an orange stick in nail care treatments.
5 What is the purpose of cuticle moisturising cream?

A selection of nail tools

A range of nail lotions and creams

167

Consult, plan and prepare for nail services with clients (3)

Client consultation

A client consultation must be carried out before a manicure or a pedicure, just as for any other salon treatment. There are many reasons why a client may book a nail care treatment and it is not only clients with good nails and surrounding skin who come to the salon for this treatment. Consulting with your client will allow you to find out what she would like and to decide, based on the condition of the client's nails and skin, how to go about your treatment.

The consultation involves the following three stages:

- questioning and recording information
- visual analysis
- manual analysis.

Questioning

Here are some of the reasons why clients come to a beauty salon for nail treatments. Remember that men may also come to the salon for a male manicure or pedicure.

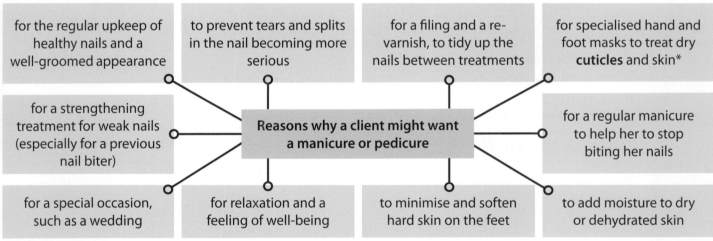

for the regular upkeep of healthy nails and a well-groomed appearance

to prevent tears and splits in the nail becoming more serious

for a filing and a re-varnish, to tidy up the nails between treatments

for specialised hand and foot masks to treat dry **cuticles** and skin*

for a strengthening treatment for weak nails (especially for a previous nail biter)

Reasons why a client might want a manicure or pedicure

for a regular manicure to help her to stop biting her nails

for a special occasion, such as a wedding

for relaxation and a feeling of well-being

to minimise and soften hard skin on the feet

to add moisture to dry or dehydrated skin

* These are not covered in Level 1

Reasons for manicures and pedicures

You need to ask to ask this information of your client to help you understand what she needs. For hand treatments, it is also important to ask about the client's lifestyle and job. This will help you to understand how much the client uses her hands and will tell you whether she is able to grow her nails long or needs to keep them short.

Visual analysis

This is when you look at the client's hands or feet, nails, skin colour and texture. It involves a thorough look at the nails and surrounding skin to find out information such as condition and strength of the nails and the condition of the skin and **cuticles**, as well as looking for anything that looks like a contra-indication.

Manual analysis

This will be carried out after completion of the paper-based part of the consultation, in which you take down client details and carry out a first visual study. You will need to clean the client's hands or feet and nails as well as your own hands by wiping over with a skin and nail cleaner or a hygienic spray. When you have done this you will be able to touch the client's hands or feet and nails in order to check them for the condition of nails, cuticles and skin, and any contra-indications and conditions.

This should be done in good light so that you are able to see well the nail and skin condition and texture. You must also write down what you see and feel on the client's record card.

Assessing the condition of a client's hands: a checklist

1 Examine the front and the backs of the hands.

2 Look at the colour and texture of the skin – is it tanned or light? Is the skin thin or thickened?

3 Are the hands soft and smooth or are they rough and chapped?

4 Does the skin show any signs of infection such as swelling, pus or lifting of the **nail plate**?

5 Are there cracks and breaks in the skin or redness around the **cuticles**?

6 Look at the skin between the fingers – are there any signs of dryness?

Assessing the condition of a client's feet: a checklist

1 Examine the top and underneath of the feet, looking carefully at the condition of the skin on the heels.

2 Look at the colour and texture of the skin – is it tanned or light? Is the skin thin or thickened?

3 Are the feet soft and smooth or are they rough and chapped?

4 Does the skin show any signs of infection such as swelling, pus or lifting of the **nail plate**?

5 Are there cracks and breaks in the skin or redness around the **cuticles**?

6 Look at the skin between the toes – are there any signs of dryness or moisture which could be an indication of athlete's foot, a fungal infection?

Assessing the condition of a client's nails: a checklist

1 What shape are the nails?

2 What length are the nails? Are they long or short? Have they been picked or bitten?

3 Are the nails healthy – strong, pink, shiny and flexible? Are they unhealthy – yellow, brittle, weak and thin?

4 Do the nails show any signs of nail diseases or disorders?

5 Is there any lifting of the nails, which could suggest nail disease or fungal infection?

6 Are the cuticles hard and overgrown, red and inflamed or smooth and even?

7 Have the cuticles grown along the nail plate?

8 Are there any **hangnails**?

Consult, plan and prepare for nail services with clients (4)

Contra-indications

A contra-indication is a condition that makes or could make a client unsuitable for a treatment. It could be unsafe to treat a client with a contra-indication. At Level 1 you are not responsible for deciding whether or not a client has a contra-indication, but you must be aware of them and be able to recognise the signs so that you can tell a senior therapist if you notice anything unusual.

Whatever level of experience therapists have, they are not qualified to diagnose medical conditions. You may have an idea of what medical condition a client may have, but the appropriate action is to refer them to their GP. You must also make sure that you do not cause the client alarm or embarrassment by talking loudly about a contra-indication so that other people may hear.

Look out for the following contra-indications. You should also look out for **athlete's foot** (which is a type of ringworm) and **verrucas** when you inspect your client's feet before a pedicure.

Warts

Ringworm

Scabies

Cuts and abrasions

Swelling and inflammation

Damaged nails

Discoloured nails

Overgrown cuticles

 Top tip

Always ask a senior member of staff to double check that you have not overlooked any infection or problem.

Get up and go!

Find as many photos of nail contra-indications as you can on the Internet. Google Images is a good place to start.

? Memory jogger

1 What is a contra-indication?

2 Why must you not diagnose a condition?

3 Name two contra-indications you may find on the feet.

4 Name two contra-indications you may find on the hands and nails.

It is a legal requirement to record client's answers to questions during the consultation, so make sure that you write everything down. For example, if a client became allergic to a product or treatment, you would have proof that you asked her questions about this.

Consult, plan and prepare for nail services with clients (5)

Recording information

Once you have completed a full consultation and before you start any treatment, you will need to record the answers and information on the client's record card. You will need to record what the client tells you about her wishes and nail care routine, and also your own observations from the visual and manual analyses. When you have completed the treatment, you will need to complete the card.

MANICURE/PEDICURE CONSULTATION CARD

Date 16/11/10   Name Jon Bomero

Address Westbrook, St Giles Road,   Date of birth 23/06/09
        Tonmouth GR7 4EL

Telephone Number (H) (01121) 556600   (W) (01121) 818120

Condition of Hands/Feet/Nails on Inspection

Hands – dry and chapped

Nails – cuticles dry and overgrown. Nails thick and stong

Contra-Indications/Conditions

None

Products Used

Simply Men manicure range

Product Sales

Homecare Advice

Carry out a salt and oil rub to help remove dry skin but avoid any
chapped areas. Use moisturiser daily.

Comments

Removed excess cuticles, buffed nails.

Advised client to return monthly.

Client Signature

Record Of Treatments

Date	Treatment	Therapist
13/01/10	Manicure	S Jones
16/11/10	Manicure	Nadia Hoffmann

A typical consultation card for a manicure or pedicure treatment

You will need to record the following.

- Client's contact details – name, address and telephone numbers. Make sure that you write down both the client's first name and surname, the postcode and a work or mobile telephone number as well as a home number. This will help to avoid confusion if you have more than one client with that surname, and will mean that you will be able to get hold of the client no matter where he or she is if you need to contact them at short notice to let them know about a change in appointment time.

- The client's wishes and information about their job and lifestyle.

- The condition of nail and hands or feet when inspected.

- Any allergies.

- Any contra-indications.

- The products used during the treatment:
  - write down any extra products, apart from the products you would always use in a manicure or pedicure, that you use on the client, such as nail strengtheners and ridge fillers
  - you should also list the varnish colour you use in case the client asks for the same colour the next time she comes to the salon.

- Advice given to the client:
  - what advice did you give your client on how they could improve the condition of their hands and nails?
  - when did you advise her to return for another salon treatment?
- Any products you sell to the client.
- Any other comments:
  - what were the results of the manicure?
  - have you any advice to other therapists? Include whatever you think may be useful to you or another therapist in the future.
- Record of treatments:
  - the date
  - the type of manicure
  - the therapist's name
  - any extra notes that could be useful for the future.

Client's consent

You must always get your client to sign the consultation to agree for the nail treatment to go ahead – this is called giving consent.

Treating a minor

If your client is under the age of 16 a parent or guardian must be present throughout the treatment and they (the parent or guardian) must sign the consultation card to give consent for the treatment to take place.

Preparing the client

Once your work area is set up, you can collect your client and ask her to sit down so that you can prepare her. The first thing you should do is wash your hands. Then place a towel over any clothing that could become marked by water or the nail care products.

Remove any items of jewellery, dress rings, bracelets, ankle bracelets and toe rings. Once you have carried out the consultation, you can help your client into the manicure or pedicure chair, making sure her position is comfortable for both of you.

Before you begin the nail manicure treatment: a checklist

1 Make a quick check of your workplace preparation.
2 Wash your hands.
3 Remove both your own and your client's watch and jewellery.
4 Protect the client's clothing.
5 Carry out a consultation.
6 Assess the condition of your client's hands and nails.
7 Check for contra-indications.

>> **Get up and go!**

Take a photo of your fully prepared work area. Include it in your portfolio to show a good set up.

? **Memory jogger**

1 Why is it important to record the answers your client gives you during consultation?
2 List four things that should be recorded on a client record card.
3 What age is a minor?

Carry out nail services (1)

Before you carry out any nail treatment, it is very important for you to understand the structure, parts and functions of the nail. Pages 210–211 of the Anatomy and physiology section of this book contain all the information you need to know.

Nail shapes

Nail shapes vary from one client to another. The natural nail shape usually mirrors the line of the **cuticle** (see the diagrams of the different nail shapes).

When shaping nails, you need to think about the following:

- the shape of the existing nail – you cannot change the natural shape of the nail, you can only improve it
- the client's lifestyle and job – for example, is she or he sporty or do they do manual work, in which case are long fingernails really practical? In the case of toenails, if the client does a lot of running, they should be short so that they don't become squashed up in trainers which could result in bruised nails
- what the client wants – clients usually have a good idea of how they want their nails to look and what needs doing. Alternatively, they may be going somewhere special and want them painted a certain colour to match an outfit
- the shape of the cuticles – when shaping the nails, follow the cuticle line for a natural look, unless the client wishes to follow the current fashion in nail shapes.

Fingernail shapes

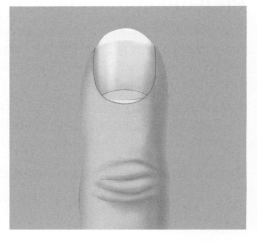

Oval

This all-purpose nail shape flatters and softens the appearance of the hands. It makes the fingers look longer. It is also quite hardwearing against breakage because of its smooth edges and flexible shape.

Round

This is also a very practical nail shape. It is hardwearing, strong and neat. However, it is not very flattering as it does not help to make the fingers look longer.

Square

This is a very good shape if the nails are short and the fingers quite long. This shape is also less likely to break because the nail wall provides good support for the sides of the nails. It is therefore ideal for people who do **manual labour**, such as typists, medical staff and cleaners. However, it is not a good shape on short fingers, as it can make them appear even shorter.

Pointed

Some clients prefer this nail shape as they believe it makes their nails look longer. However, it is best to advise against this shape as the nails are filed to a point from the corners to the tip. The corners where the free edge starts are the **stress points** of the nails – the nails have no support from the nail wall so can easily weaken and split.

Toenail shapes

These tend to be naturally square or rounded. When shaping them during a pedicure, they must be filed or cut straight across making sure you don't shape them into the corners as this can cause ingrown toenails.

 Get up and go!

Look at the different fingernail shapes on your fellow students. Which are the most common?

? Memory jogger

1 List three fingernail shapes.

2 How should you shape a toenail?

3 How will you decide what shape to do the fingernails?

Carry out nail services (2)

Manicures

A manicure is a treatment carried out to improve and beautify the condition of the hands and nails. It takes about 30–45 minutes to complete and its aims are to:

- clean and shape the nails
- care for the **cuticles**
- soften dry skin on the hands
- relax the muscles in the hand and arm
- give a healthy shine to the nails.

A manicure includes the following:

- a hand and nail inspection – to check the condition of the hands and for any problem areas
- filing and **bevelling** – to neaten the nails and remove splits and catches
- soaking – to soften the skin for cuticle work
- cuticle work – to push back and neaten the cuticles
- massage – to moisturise the skin, improve blood flow and relax the client
- **buffing** – to smooth ridges, give a healthy shine and improve the blood flow
- painting – to beautify the nails by adding colour and shine.

After a manicure, the nails should look naturally polished or perfectly painted. The skin on the hands and around the cuticles should be soft and smooth.

Step-by-step manicure

This diagram illustrates the stages involved in a manicure.

Top tips ✓

- Explain to your client what you are doing as you go along and why, because it is important to keep the client informed.
- Chat to the client about her wishes for today's treatment. Remember that these can change from one week to the next, so remember to check each time.

Summary of steps in a manicure

Removing nail varnish

When you have carried out your consultation and prepared your client for her manicure, your first step is to clean the client's nails and remove any varnish she might have on.

 Top tips

- A fresh piece of cotton wool should be used for each nail, because once there is a build-up of dissolved varnish on the cotton wool ball, it is not as good at removing varnish.
- Nail varnish tends to stain around the cuticle and nail fold, so use a covered orange stick dipped in nail varnish remover to remove the varnish from these areas.

Filing and bevelling

Do not saw in both directions, as this will cause the nail to split. Use the file at a 45° angle to the nail and file from one side of the nail to the centre, then file from the other side to the centre.

45° angle

File the nail at a 45° angle

Side-to-centre action

Top tip

If the nails are very long and need cutting, this is best done after they have been softened by soaking in water. Cutting hard, dry nails will cause the nail layers to separate and the nails to split.

Cuticle work

Cuticle cream both softens the **cuticles** so that they are easier to push back and moisturises dry skin and nails. It also acts as a nail shampoo and will help get rid of staining or stubborn dirt. Place any loose bits of cuticle or dirt on a tissue and throw it away afterwards.

Cuticle remover must be wiped off thoroughly, otherwise it may carry on working and could cause soreness.

 Top tip

Scarf nail is the name for fine wisps of nail that stick out after soaking. They are very flimsy and thin, like a scarf.

Carry out nail services (3)

Massage and moisturise

Moisturising softens and smoothes the skin and is a perfect finish to a manicure. The moisturiser or massage cream is applied and rubbed into the skin using rubbing and kneading movements (see page 187).

A simple massage routine is to start with lighter strokes that become deeper. Begin with the arm up to the elbow, then move down to the hands and the fingers. The hand and arm massage routine should take about five to ten minutes to complete on both hands.

After you have carried out a massage using a rich moisturising or massage cream there may still be some cream on the nail. If it remains on the nail, the nail varnish will not go on smoothly and will not dry properly. If you do manage to paint nail varnish on the nails, the varnish will soon peel off once you have finished. It is therefore very important that you degrease the nails thoroughly with nail varnish remover following the massage.

 Top tip

For Level 1, it is not necessary for you to follow a set massage routine using all the movements. However, it is important that you carry out some sort of massage routine that is relaxing to the client.

 Get ahead

Plan a six-week treatment programme for one of your friends, family or clients which is aimed at improving the skin and nails of their hands or feet. Your plan should include full details of what you will do during each of the six weeks and how each of the treatments will help them.

Buffing

If a client chooses not to have her nails painted, offer to buff them for her. This will improve the circulation in her nails and polish them, leaving a healthy, natural shine.

 Top tip

Do not rub while **buffing** as this will create heat, which can be painful as well as damaging to the layers of the nail. Do about four to six strokes on each nail in a downward direction. Do not be tempted to do any more strokes.

Painting

 Top tip

If the client wants a varnish, now is the time to ask her to put all her jewellery back on, to put on her jacket or coat, and to get her car keys out of her handbag. You should also politely ask if she would like to pay for the manicure before you paint her nails, explaining about the drying time of varnishes.

Nail varnish should be painted on in a **methodical** way. Here is a guide to show you how best to do this.

Painting your client's nails

1 Make sure that your client's nails are very clean – there should be no dirt or grease on them.

2 Prepare a cotton wool-coated orange stick by soaking it in nail vanish remover. This is in case you make a mistake while painting or to clean off any varnish around the **cuticle**. It is better to remove the nail varnish straight away, because wet nail varnish is easier to remove than dry nail varnish.

3 Paint the nails. While painting, support the client's hand while holding the nail varnish bottle and complete the strokes with your other hand.

Painting the nails

a   b   c   d

When painting the nails:

a begin with one central application

b then apply the varnish to the right

c then apply the varnish to the left

d go over the whole nail to smooth the varnish.

Carry out nail services (4)

Painting tips

Do:

- make sure that you have enough varnish on the brush to do the whole nail
- paint thinly
- use only a few strokes
- leave a small gap at the base of the nail before the **cuticle**
- hold the bottle while you paint.

Don't:

- overload the brush with paint, as it will drip down and flood the nail with too much varnish
- paint thickly, as it will take too long to dry
- use too many brush strokes, as the finish will be lumpy and uneven
- paint right up to the cuticle, as the varnish will seep into the skin and look messy
- dip the brush in a bottle that is not held, as it could fall over and spill varnish.

While painting, leave a small gap at the base of the nail before the cuticle

To prevent smudging, follow the finger rotation method

Start
1 Replace client's jewellery and take payment
2 Choose colour
3 Degrease nails
4 Apply base coat
5 Apply two coats of varnish
6 If cream varnish, apply top coat
7 Apply nail dry
Finish

Summary of steps involved in painting nails

Polish profile

Base coats

These can be clear or pale coloured. They are applied to the **nail plate** before varnish to:

- smooth the nail
- cut down on staining from bright coloured varnishes
- help prevent early chipping or the colour wearing off.

Top coats

These are usually clear and are used to:

- give a high shine to the coloured nails
- help to make the varnish last longer.

Some top coats also have an added ingredient which helps to speed up the drying time.

Ridge-filling base coats

These are usually pale in colour and thicker than normal base coats. If a client has a very uneven nail plate with ridges or dips, the ridge filler will help to smooth the surface of the nail.

Nail hardeners

These are clear varnishes but have ingredients that are meant to provide the nails with a tough coating.

Nail strengtheners

These are usually clear and have nourishing and strengthening ingredients to help weak nails grow.

Cream nail varnish

Cream nail varnish is better for nails with many ridges and dents, as it does not show them up. The basic rule with cream nail varnish is:

- base coat
- two coats of cream varnish
- top coat.

Pearlised nail varnish

Pearlised nail varnish contains ingredients that give it a shimmery look. However, it shows up uneven surfaces in the nail plate, so should not be used on nails that are not healthy looking and smooth. With pearlised varnishes, the basic rule is:

- base coat
- two or three coats of varnish
- no top coat.

Solvents

Although not a varnish product, solvents are used to dissolve nail varnishes from furniture and clothes if they have been spilled, although this process is not always completely successful. However, the main use of solvent is to thin out nail varnishes when they become thick and sticky. A few drops in a bottle of varnish when shaken gives new life to a varnish, leaving it as thin as when it was first opened.

Top tip

Base coats and top coats can be used if a client wants a clear varnish instead of a colour varnish.

Get ahead

Investigate the ingredients found in nail varnishes and how the ingredients in different ones vary. For example, what ingredients are different in a pearlised nail varnish and a hardener? Make a poster or leaflet to show the ingredients in each product.

Carry out nail services (5)

The ingredients in nail varnish

It may help you to know more about the main ingredients in nail varnish and what they do. This information is presented in the table below.

Ingredient	Purpose
Nitrocellulose and resin	Carry the colour
Ethyl acetate	Helps speed up the drying time
Plasticiser	Makes the varnish flexible
Pigments	Gives colour
Bentonite clay	Stops colour separating

Choosing a nail varnish colour

Nail varnish comes in many colours. As a beauty therapist, you need to be aware of a few things before you can help your client choose the best nail varnish colour.

The length of the nails

Very bright colours on short or bitten nails will only draw attention to them and make the nails look shorter than they are.

The condition of the cuticles

Red-looking **cuticles** can look worse if the nails are painted in a bright or pearlised varnish. Pale and neutral colours in a cream varnish look better.

The client's home life and job

If a client has a job that could cause the nails to chip quite quickly, it is best to have a colour that is not going to show the odd little chip too much.

The client's skin colour

Orange, peach or beige colours show up the bluish colour in skin with poor circulation. Pinks clash with reddish skin tones.

The condition and smoothness of the nails

Pearlised varnish will show up any imperfections such as dents and ridges, so use a ridge-filling base coat and a cream varnish.

The size of the fingernails

Dark colours make the nails look smaller.

Get up and go!

Make a nail varnish chart that can be showed to the client. Get a piece of white card and place blobs of different coloured nail varnish on it. This will take a while to dry, perhaps even overnight. When the blobs are dry, label them all with the names of the varnishes. Keep this card in your portfolio and when doing your nail treatments allow the client to choose from the colours at the start.

Specialised treatments

Basic manicures and pedicures can be added to so that they become specialised. Here are some examples:

- exfoliating treatments – a rough cream is massaged into the feet and ball of the foot in circular movements to remove dead dry skin. It also improves the circulation and appearance of the skin

- foot or hand treatment mask – this can be applied at different stages of the treatment depending on the requirements. The hands or feet are then put into thermal booties to help the mask work better. The treatment improves the circulation, removes dead skin cells and softens the skin

- paraffin wax – a heated wax is applied to the hands or feet with a brush. The effects stimulate the circulation, help aches and pains and soften the skin.

Salon life

Penny had done a brilliant job of a manicure on Mrs Aziz but realised that she had not asked her client to choose a varnish colour at the start. Penny got the box of varnish colours and asked her client to choose a colour. Mrs Aziz chose the midnight black but, unfortunately, when Penny tried to open it, it was stuck.

Penny ran it under warm water and eventually managed to open the bottle top. The trouble was it was sticky and thick, and Penny knew that it would not go on very well, so she poured in some nail varnish remover and it thinned out really well.

Penny started to paint the fingernails but halfway through the varnish started to thicken again and it went on in a very lumpy and uneven way which made Mrs Aziz complain.

Is nail varnish remover a good way to thin a nail varnish? If not, what would be the best way to do this?

Why did the varnish start to thicken again?

Was the salon to blame in any way?

Carry out nail services (6)

Step-by-step manicure

1　Wipe over the front and back of your client's hands with antiseptic. Carry out a consultation and check for contra-indications. Protect your client's sleeves with tissue.

2　Right hand. Soak a clean ball of cotton wool with nail varnish remover. Hold on to the **nail plate** briefly, then wipe downwards to remove the dissolved varnish. Cover an orange stick with cotton wool, dip the end in nail varnish remover, and use this to go around the cuticle and nail fold.

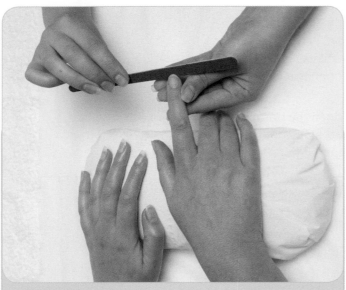

3　Right hand. File the nails using the fine side of the emery board.

4　Right hand. Turn the emery board lengthways to the nail and very gently buff the tip of the nail with the fine side. This action is called bevelling. Bevelling seals the free edges of the nail, which prevents them from splitting and peeling back.

5 Right hand. Use a clean spatula to scoop out a small amount of cuticle cream. Dip a covered orange stick into the cream and apply it to the centre of the cuticles on each nail. Massage in the cuticle cream in a circular action so that it covers the nails and cuticles.

6 Place your client's right hand in a bowl containing warm soapy water. Repeat steps 2–6 on the client's left hand.

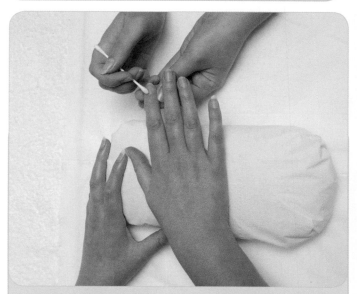

7 Take your client's right hand out of the water. Place the client's left hand in the water.

8 Dry your client's hand thoroughly, pushing the cuticles back with the towel. The senior therapist will then use a clean covered orange stick or cotton bud to apply cuticle remover to the cuticles and underneath the free edge. They will push back gently using circular actions, and clean under the free edge.

Carry out nail services (7)

Step-by-step manicure

9 The senior therapist may need to ease away any excess cuticle with a cuticle knife. If there are any **hangnails** or loose bits of skin on the cuticles, she will also need to use the cuticle nippers to remove them.

10 Remove the last traces of cuticle remover with a damp piece of cotton wool. Finally push back the treated cuticle with a rubber hoof stick.

11 Take the client's left hand out of the water. Repeat steps 8–10 on the client's left hand. Tidy up the free edges of the nails on both hands with the emery board because very fine wisps of nail may have appeared, called **scarf nail**.

12 Using a spatula, place a small amount of massage cream or hand cream into the palm of your hands. Stroke the cream on to the skin of your client's arms using smooth upward effleurage movements.

13 Massage using a variety of flowing effleurage and gentle kneading (petrissage) movements.

14 Finally, use petrissage techniques on the backs of both hands. Hand massage should take about five minutes.

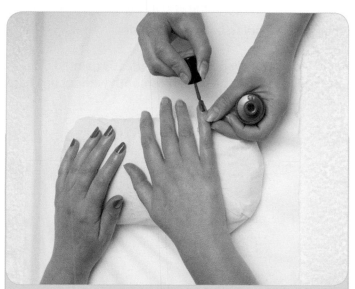

15 If you are going to buff your client's nails, do so at this point. Otherwise proceed with painting your client's nails. Go over the nail with nail varnish remover to degrease the **nail plate**, as you did at the start of your manicure. Paint the nails, following the routine described on pages 179 to 180.

16 Check the finished result – the paint or polish completes the look.

Carry out nail services (8)

Pedicures

Pedicures are similar to manicures except that they are carried out on the feet instead of the hands. They improve the condition of the feet and toenails and take about an hour to complete. The aims of a pedicure are to:

- clean and shape the nails
- care for the cuticles
- soften dry skin on the feet, especially the heels
- relax the muscles in the leg and foot
- give a healthy shine to the nails.

A pedicure includes the following:

- a foot and toenail inspection – to check the condition of the skin on the feet and look for any problem areas
- filing and bevelling – to neaten the nails and remove splits and catches
- soaking – to soften the skin for cuticle work
- cuticle work – to push back and neaten the cuticles
- hard skin removal – using a foot file, rasp or **pumice stone**
- massage – to moisturise the skin, improve blood flow and relax the client
- buffing – to smooth ridges, give a healthy shine and improve the blood flow
- painting – to beautify the nails by adding colour and shine.

After a pedicure, the nails should look naturally polished or perfectly painted. The skin on the feet and around the cuticles should be soft and smooth without any hard skin or cracks on the heels.

Step-by-step pedicure

Start

1 Preparation and consultation

2 Check for contra-indications

3 Remove varnish

4 File and bevel

5 Cuticle massage cream

6 Soak

7 Cut toenails if necessary

8 Cuticle work

9 Rough skin remover

10 Massage and moisturise

11 Painting or buffing

Finish

? Memory jogger

1 List three nail-painting tips.

2 What is the purpose of buffing?

3 Why should you wipe over the nails with nail varnish remover before painting them?

4 What is a solvent?

5 What type of nail varnish is better for nails with ridges and dents?

Summary of steps in a pedicure

Carry out nail services (9)

Step-by-step pedicure

1 Wipe over the front and back of your client's feet with antiseptic. Carry out a consultation and check for contra-indications. Protect your client's trousers or skirt with a towel and couch roll for protection against water splashes and creams and lotions.

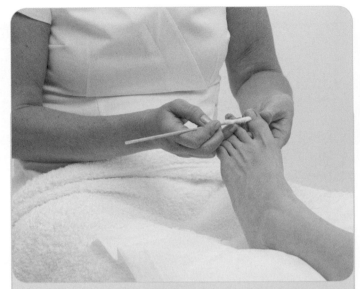

2 First foot. Soak a clean ball of cotton wool with nail varnish remover. Hold onto the **nail plate** briefly, then wipe downwards to remove the dissolved varnish. Cover an orange stick with cotton wool, dip the end into some nail varnish remover, and use this to go around the cuticle and nail fold.

3 If the toenails don't need cutting, (the senior therapist will cut them after they have been soaked) file the nails on the first foot using the coarse side of the emery board, unless the toenails are thin, in which case you will need to use the fine side.

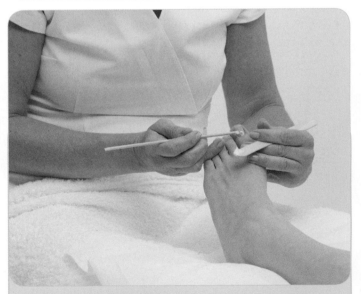

4 First foot. Turn the emery board lengthways and very gently buff the tip of the nail with the fine side. Use a clean spatula to scoop out some cuticle cream. Dip a covered orange stick into the cream and apply it to the centre of the cuticles on each nail. Massage in the cream in a circular action.

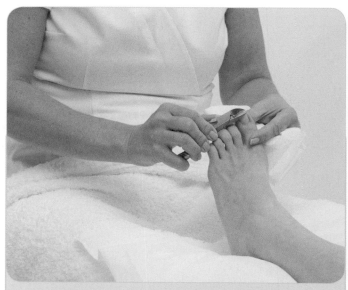

5 Place your client's first foot in the bowl or foot spa containing warm soapy water. On the client's second foot, repeat steps 2–4.

6 Take the client's first foot out of the water. Place the client's second foot in the water. Dry the client's first foot and nails thoroughly using a towel, pushing back the cuticles with the towel as you go. The senior therapist may now cut the toenails if necessary.

7 On the first foot, the senior therapist will use a clean covered orange stick to apply cuticle remover to the cuticles of each nail and underneath the free edge. When she has finished, take the orange stick, push back gently using circular actions, and clean under the free edge.

8 The senior therapist may need to ease away any excess cuticle with a cuticle knife. If there are any **hangnails** or loose bits of skin on the cuticles she will also need to use the cuticle nippers to remove them.

Carry out nail services (10)

Step-by-step pedicure

9 Remove the last traces of cuticle remover with damp cotton wool. Throw it away. Push back the treated cuticle with a rubber hoof stick. Take the client's other foot out of the water. Dry the foot and nails thoroughly, pushing back the cuticles with the towel. Repeat steps 7–9 on this foot.

10 Tidy up the free edges of the nails on both feet with the emery board because very fine wisps of nail may have appeared, called **scarf nail**.

11 You may apply rough skin remover to the areas that need attention, most commonly the ball of the foot, the heel and side of the big toe. The senior therapist can use a foot rasp here if the skin is very rough.

12 Using a spatula, place a small amount of massage cream into the palm of your hands. Stroke the cream on to the skin of your client's feet and legs using smooth upward effleurage movements. The muscles in the lower leg are quite strong and a deep massage will help to relax them.

13 Massage using a variety of flowing effleurage and gentle kneading (petrissage) movements.

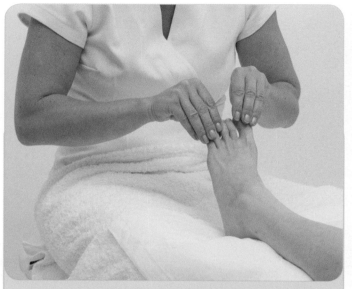

14 Finally, use petrissage techniques on the toes of both feet. Foot and leg massage should take about five minutes.

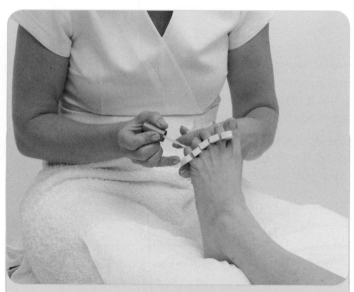

15 If you are going to buff your client's nails, do so at this point. Otherwise proceed with painting your client's nails. Go over the nail with nail varnish remover to degrease the **nail plate**. Paint the nails, following the routine described on pages 179 to 180.

16 Check the finished result – the paint or polish completes the look.

Provide aftercare advice

Checking client satisfaction

When the whole manicure or pedicure and painting treatment is complete, you will need to check that the client is happy with the result. The easiest and most obvious way is to ask her. If there is anything that she is not happy about, then it is your job to put it right with the help of your supervisor.

If the client is satisfied with her treatment, you will then need to check that the finished effect meets the senior therapist's approval and that you completed the treatment within a commercially viable time (see page 89).

Next, you will need to complete the record card, adding anything about the treatment and products used as well as any information about how the treatment went.

 Top tips

- Leaving your work area clean and tidy ready for the next treatment is essential. Replace all furniture, put away products, replace dirty laundry, wipe surfaces, re-sterilise tools and get clean disinfectant.
- If the client is happy with her manicure and likes the products that you have used, it would be a good idea to ask her if she would like to look at the products on sale. Handy take-home packs are a good selling point, as they allow the client to continue with her nail care at home.

Male nails

Salon treatments for men are becoming more popular. Manicures and pedicures are especially popular as men like to look well groomed. The basic routine is the same – the only difference is that men tend to have their nails buffed instead of painted. Some men, however, do like a clear coat of varnish to give their nails a healthy shine.

Men who do manual jobs, such as car mechanics and builders, may have untidy and tough **cuticles**. They may also have a lot of staining to the nails, cuticles and under the free edge, so make sure that you have a very good cuticle remover.

 Top tip

For men with tough and stained cuticles, apply the cuticle remover generously, then leave it on for a couple of minutes. This will give the active ingredient sufficient time to bleach out the stains and prepare the cuticles for further treatment.

Homecare advice

After the manicure or pedicure, you should advise your client on how best to look after her nails so that they remain in the best condition.

The following list is good homecare advice for clients.

1   Wear rubber gloves when washing up or using strong cleaning products.

2   Keep hand cream by the sink and apply it after washing up. Wear hand cream at night.

3   Wear gardening gloves – don't use bare hands in the garden.

4   Don't use your nails as tools as this will weaken or break them.

5   Rinse off harsh products from the skin immediately as they could cause a rash or soreness.

6   Remove rings before washing so that soap does not build up under the rings and irritate the skin.

7   If there is a split on the nail, bevel it gently as soon as possible. (You may have to show your client what to do.)

8   Keep an emery board with you at all times so that you can smooth away any catch in the nail instantly.

9   Apply a top coat of polish over painted nails every other day, to make the varnish last longer.

10 Don't be tempted to pick dry **cuticles** – use a rich cream to soften them.

11 Always use a base coat under varnish to protect the nails from becoming stained.

12 Try to make time for a manicure every two weeks.

13 Try to make time for a pedicure every month.

14 Change socks or tights daily.

15 Make sure that footwear fits properly and is not tight.

16 Always file nails straight across.

17 Avoid wearing high heels for long periods of time.

18 Apply moisturiser to the feet after showering and having a bath.

≫ Get up and go!

Take photos of your own or your partner's hands and feet before and after a treatment. Use these to make a poster advertising the benefits of a manicure and pedicure. Remember to make it colourful and eye-catching.

? Memory jogger

1   List four pieces of aftercare advice you could give to a client after a manicure.

2   List four pieces of aftercare advice you could give to a client after a pedicure.

Getting ready for assessment

Evidence requirements

You will be observed by your assessor on at least three occasions, one of which must be on the feet.

What you must cover during your practical assessments

Ranges

In your candidate log book you will have a list of ranges that you must cover during your assessment. These ranges cover:

1 consultation techniques

2 nail finish

3 advice.

From the range you must show that you:

- have used all consultation techniques
- have applied three of the four types of nail finishes
- have provided all advice.

It is good practice to cover as many ranges as possible during each assessment. This will prevent you having to take too many additional assessments because there are many ranges that you have not managed to cover.

Performance criteria

What you must demonstrate during a practical observation by your tutor:

- preparation for nail treatments
- an assessment of the condition of skin and nails
- good communication skills
- basic nail care treatments
- checking the client is happy with the treatment and finished effect
- giving aftercare advice to the client
- leaving the work area in a suitable condition.

Throughout your observations you will also need to make sure that you pay attention to health, safety and hygiene throughout, as well as presenting yourself well, so read through Unit G20 Make sure your own actions reduce risks to health and safety before any practical assessment just to refresh your memory.

Carrying out a practical treatment using unhygienic tools, or without carrying out a risk assessment of your work area to avoid accidents happening, will mean that you are not safe to do a treatment and therefore could mean that you do not pass your assessment.

What you must know

In order to pass this unit, you will need to gather evidence during the teaching and learning of this unit before your assessor observes your practical performance. You will gather this during class work and further study and will probably file it in a portfolio of evidence. This evidence will also be signed off in your candidate log book which you will be given by your assessor. This will be an official record to show that you have covered what you need to.

Salon life

During a consultation with her client, Eve realised that what the client wanted was not in her best interests. The client's nails were dry and brittle, and the cuticles were very hard and slightly inflamed with skin that had grown along the nail plate. The client wanted a basic manicure and her nails painted a bright red colour – she had brought the colour in herself.

Very politely, Eve set about advising her client that, rather than a basic manicure, her nails needed some tender care.

What homecare advice should Eve provide to the client to get her nails back into good condition?

Get up and go!

Investigate the products that you can buy to improve the condition of the nails at home. Create a poster with the pictures of the products and a brief description of what they do. Visit www.pearsonhotlinks.co.uk and search for this title for links to websites that will help you with this.

Anatomy and physiology

In this section you will find the essential anatomy and physiology that you need to know to be able to carry out face and nail treatments for Level 1 Beauty Therapy.

As a beauty therapy assistant at Level 1 it is important to have a good knowledge of anatomy and physiology as many of the treatments that you will be learning about have an effect on the functioning and systems of the body. For example, massage of the face, hands and feet will improve the circulation, relax the muscles and improve the appearance of the skin.

In this unit you will learn about:

- Anatomy and physiology for facial treatments and make-up
- Anatomy and physiology for nail treatments.

Here are some key terms you will meet in this unit:

Sebum – an oily substance secreted from sebaceous glands

Physiology – bodily processes

Impurities – dirt and germs that can cause bad health and poor skin

Anatomy – framework, structure of the body, e.g. bones and muscles

Functions – purpose, job

Inflamed – red and swollen, possibly because of an infection

Elasticity – stretchiness

Toxins – poisons

Cranium – the part of the skull that encloses the brain

Secretes – seeps, oozes

Nail bed – the layer of cells on which the nail plate rests

Nail grooves – deep ridges that guide the direction of nail growth

Lunula – the half moon at the base of the nail

Skull – the part of the skeleton that is found in the head

Nutrients – vitamins and minerals

Anatomy and physiology for facial treatments and make-up (1)

Knowledge of **anatomy** and **physiology** for facial treatments and make-up will help you to understand the bone structure and shape of the face, because your make-up techniques and application methods should aim to enhance the face's natural shape. Facial treatments require massage of the face, neck and shoulder, so it is important to know about the muscles underneath the skin as well as the effect of ageing on the skin and the how the skin **functions** keep it healthy.

The skin

The skin is a fascinating organ. Have a look at these facts about the largest organ of the body.

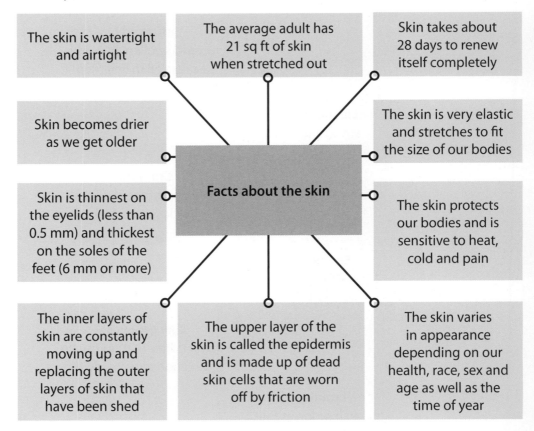

Amazing facts about the skin

The structure of the skin

The skin has three main layers:

- the epidermis
- the dermis
- the fatty layer.

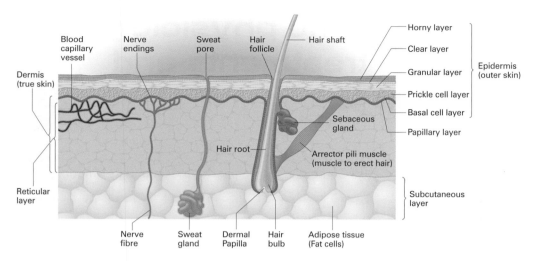

The structure of the skin

The upper layer of the skin (epidermis) is made up of five layers. Each layer has a different job to do in order to keep the skin healthy. It is not essential that you know about the five layers of skin at Level 1, but it may be useful to understand a little about them.

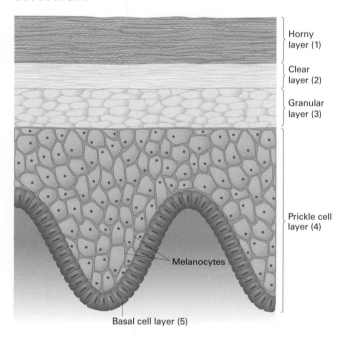

Look at the table below. You may find it easier to remember and say the English names rather than the Latin ones. It may also be helpful to know that *stratum* is the Latin word for layer.

The five layers of the epidermis

The five layers of the epidermis are as follows.

Layer	Latin name	English name
Layer 1	Stratum corneum	Horny layer
Layer 2	Stratum lucidum	Clear layer
Layer 3	Stratum granulosum	Granular layer
Layer 4	Stratum spinosum	Prickle cell layer
Layer 5	Stratum germinativum	Basal cell layer

Anatomy and physiology for facial treatments and make-up (2)

The skin

Knowing about the structure of the skin can help us to understand its **functions**.

> **» Get up and go!**
>
> Make a card game or board game that will help you to remember the parts of the skin, the functions of the skin or some facts about skin. Be adventurous and creative.
>
> Once you have created your game, play it with other students in your class. A card game could be based around the structure of the skin, with each card having the correct name of the skin layer on one side and on the other the function it has. It is up to you how you design your game, but the most important thing is that it helps you to remember things based around anatomy and physiology.

Functions of the skin

The skin does many important jobs, without which our bodies could overheat, become ill and get injured easily.

- Vitamin production – the sun's rays on the skin make vitamin D for the body. This vitamin is needed for strong bones and teeth.

- Sense and feeling – the nerve endings in our skin are very sensitive. They pick up changes in temperature or pressure, and alert us to pain. Messages are quickly sent from the nerve endings to our brain so that we can respond – for example, by stopping the source of the pain.

- Heat control – skin helps to control the temperature in our body, e.g. how hot or cold we are. When we are too hot, we begin to sweat through sweat glands in our skin, and this cools us down. When we are too cold, the muscles that are joined to the hairs in our skin cause goose pimples and we begin to shiver, which warms up the body. The correct temperature of the skin should be about 36°C.

- Absorption – the skin is able to absorb small amounts of products that are put on the skin.

- Protection – skin is like a waterproof jacket as it provides the body with protection from dirt, bacteria and injury. To keep the outer layers of skin smooth and soft and free from splits and cracks that would let germs enter, the body produces oil through the skin's pores.

- Excretion – some waste products and **toxins** are removed from the body through our sweat.

- Secretion – the skin **secretes** a substance through its pores called **sebum**, which keeps our skin smooth and supple.
- Storage – the skin stores fat and water, without which we could not survive.

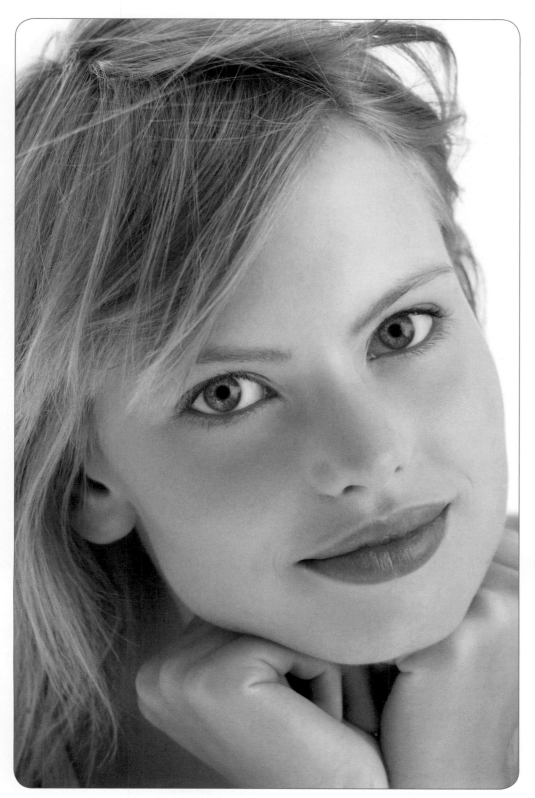

The skin does many important jobs, so make sure you look after yours

Memory jogger

1 How many layers of the epidermis are there?

A 3

B 4

C 5

D 6

2 What are the eight functions of the skin?

Anatomy and physiology for facial treatments and make-up (3)

The skin

Healthy skin

Given all of the jobs that our skin does, it is easy to understand why it is so important to look after it. The skin on our faces can reveal how healthy we are. When we are healthy our skin glows, and when we are ill the effects can be seen in the colour and condition of our faces. The skin can also reflect how we feel – when we are fed up, stressed or have an illness, the skin becomes dull and lifeless. As we get older, facial skin can reveal the sort of life we have lived.

If we have sunbathed too much	the skin will be thickened, orangey yellow and very lined
If we have smoked	the skin around the mouth will have lines from sucking on the cigarette, and the nose and cheeks may be red with broken veins from the heat and smoke of the cigarette
If we have cried or laughed a lot	the fine skin around the eyes can be very wrinkled
If we have frowned a lot	we may have deep ridges in between our eyebrows
When we are dehydrated	our skin becomes dry and flaky
When we have a temperature	the skin flushes and becomes sweaty
When we feel sick	the skin looks pale and grey
If we eat an unhealthy diet	we may have blotchy, spotty skin

How our actions affect our skin

The skin varies in appearance depending on our sex, age and race as well as changing in different seasons. Our diet, health and lifestyle also affect our skin so it is important to remember to care for it and treat it well throughout our life. Skin that is cared for well in teenage years will mean healthier and more attractive skin when you are in your 50s and 60s.

>> **Get up and go!**

Think about members of your family, both male and female, old and young. What do you notice about their skin? Write down your observations and then discuss them in groups.

Tips for healthy skin

Here are some tips for healthy skin. You may want to mention some of these in the aftercare advice you give to your clients.

Weather

Protect the skin with creams that contain a UV-filter (at least SPF 15) when in the sun and use a rich moisturiser in cold weather.

Exercise

Exercise improves the body's circulation (the blood flow around the body) which in turn improves the skin's colour and texture.

Alcohol and drugs

These cause dehydration, which dries out the skin. They also result in the body losing important **nutrients** that the skin needs to work properly.

Smoking

Smoking ages and dries out the skin, and causes tiny broken blood vessels to appear. If you don't smoke, stay away from smoky areas.

Cleansing

It is important to keep the skin clean by cleansing every day. This prevents germs from building up and causing an infection. In addition, a dirty complexion is unattractive and looks unhealthy.

Sleep

It is important that you get plenty of sleep, because when you sleep your skin rests and repairs itself.

What you eat

It is important to eat a balanced diet that includes lots of fresh fruit and vegetables, and all of the vitamins and minerals that your body needs.

Water

Drink lots of water daily – about eight glasses. Water flushes out **impurities** from the body, which helps to keep the skin clear and prevents it from drying out.

Ageing

As the skin gets older it loses moisture and **elasticity**, so it is important to take care of the skin from a young age by using moisturisers and gentle skin care.

Young skin   Mature skin

> **? Memory jogger**
>
> 1 How does exercise improve the skin's colour and texture?
> 2 As the skin ages, it loses:
>   A Elasticity
>   B Cleanliness
>   C Colour
>   D Impurities
> 3 When does your skin rest and repair itself?
>   A During the daytime
>   B During exercise
>   C After mealtimes
>   D During sleep
> 4 How does dehydration affect the skin?
>   A It makes it oily
>   B It makes it shiny
>   C It makes it flaky
>   D It makes it dirty

Anatomy and physiology for facial treatments and make-up (4)

Muscles and bones of the face and head

Underneath the skin are muscles and bones.

- The muscles allow for facial movement, and each facial muscle produces a different movement.
- The bones provide support for the muscles, and protect the brain and facial organs from injury.

The muscles and bones also give shape to the face. When carrying out make-up treatments your techniques should aim to enhance the natural shape.

Muscles

Many of the muscles found on the face are very small and attached to other muscles. For Level 1 you do not need to know the correct names and actions of the muscles, but the diagram below will help you to understand the face better when you carry out practical treatments.

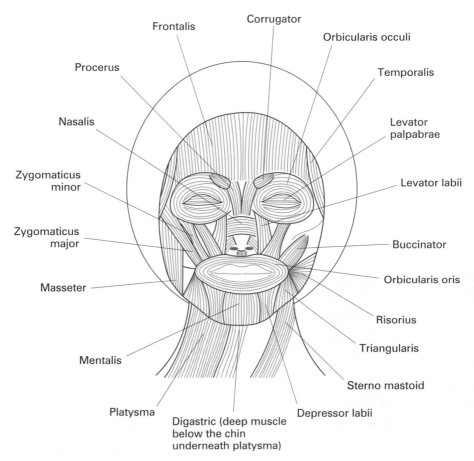

Muscles of the face and neck

When we make different facial expressions such as smiling, laughing or frowning, the muscles pull our faces into different shapes, as shown in the diagram below.

1. FRONTALIS
Amazement,
wonder,
shock

**2. ORBICULARIS
OCULI**

Deep thought

3. PROCERUS
Threatening,
unfriendliness,
anger

4. CORRUGATOR
Sadness and sorrow,
regret

**5. ZYGOMATICUS
MAJOR**
Laughter

**6. LEVATOR LABII
SUPERIORIS**
Grief, discontented

7. LEVATOR LABII
Extreme grief with
tears

**8. COMPRESSOR
NARIS**
Concentration, interest and
attention or anger and violent behaviour

**9. ORBICULARIS
ORIS**
Pouting, smoking,
kissing

**10. DEPRESSOR
ANGULIORIS**
Dislike, disapproval

**11. DEPRESSOR
LABII INFERIORIS**
Disgust

12. PLATYSMA
Anger, pain, torture
or hard work

 Get up and go!

Mould some plasticine into the shape of facial muscles using this book to guide you. Place it over a model of a skeleton.

The actions of different facial muscles in facial expressions

Get ahead

Copy the 12 facial expressions in the diagram above. See if you can work out which muscles are being used for each expression. It will help if you make faces at each other.

Anatomy and physiology for facial treatments and make-up (5)

The bones of the head, otherwise known as the **skull**, keep the muscles in place and protect the brain and other parts of the head from injury. The skull is made up of the **cranium** and the lower jaw (mandible). There are 22 bones in the skull in total. Eight of these make up the cranium, as shown in the table below.

Bone	Position
1 x ethmoid bone	At the roof of the nose
1 x frontal bone	Forms the front of the cranium, forehead and upper eye sockets
1 x occipital bone	At the back and lower part of the cranium
2 x parietal bones	At the back and top of the cranium
1 x sphenoid bone	At the base of the cranium, in front of the temporal bones
2 x temporal bones	At the side, around the ears

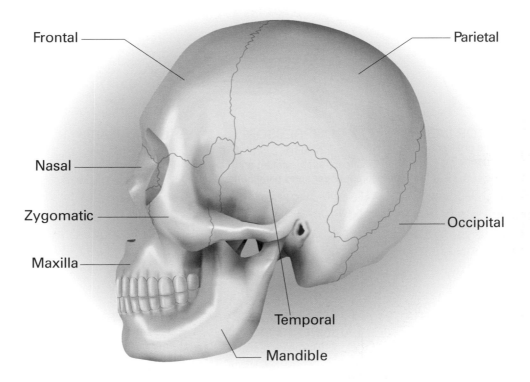

The bones of the skull

The face

The bones of the face also protect the soft tissues inside the head. The face is made up of 14 bones. The seven main ones are shown in the table below.

Bone	Position
1 x mandible	This is the lower jaw and is the only moving bone in the face. It enables movement of the mouth for chewing and talking
2 x maxillae	These form the upper jaw, most of the side wall of the nose and the front part of the soft palate (the top of the mouth)
2 x nasal bones	These form the bridge (upper part) of the nose
2 x zygomatic bones	These form the cheekbones

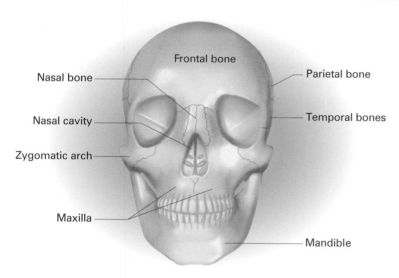

The bones of the face

How the bones affect facial shape

The photo below shows a person with prominent (noticeable) cheekbones. The bones that create this are called the zygomatic bones and some people have less prominent ones than others. The line of the chin and jaw is decided by the mandible bone. The shape of the nose is decided by the nasal bones. All of the bones in our face and head shape us.

The bones of the face affect its shape

>> **Get up and go!**

Take photographs of each other's faces, print them off and draw the bones on the photograph. Activities like this that are practical will help you to remember information better.

? **Memory jogger**

1 How many bones are there in the face?
   A 5
   B 8
   C 14
   D 22

2 Which bone forms the forehead?

3 Which bone might you apply cheek colour to?
   A Maxilla
   B Mandible
   C Zygomatic
   D Occipital

4 Name one function of bone.

Anatomy and physiology for nail treatments (1)

In the same way that knowing about the bones and structure of the face is helpful for facial treatments, understanding the structure of the hand and nails is useful knowledge for nail treatments. The structure of the nail and how to keep it healthy is valuable information to pass on to clients, whereas knowledge of the muscles and structure of the hand is useful for massage therapies.

The nails

The structure of nails

The nails grow from the ends of the fingers and toes. The nail plate is a hard, rectangular and curved structure made up of flat layers of cells. It covers and protects the sensitive fingertips and **nail bed**. When healthy a nail should be pink, smooth and flexible with a white free edge that shows no signs of flaking or splitting. The cuticle should not be dry, rough or **inflamed**.

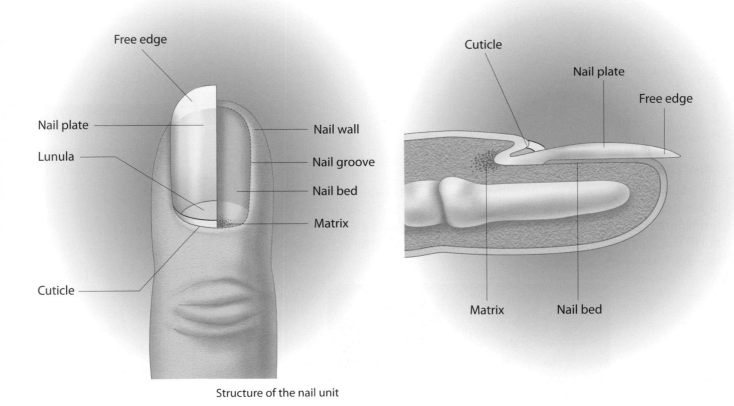

Structure of the nail unit

Parts and functions of the nail

Matrix

The **matrix** is the only living part of the nail. Its function is to grow and replace the cells that form the nail. The quality, strength and health of the nail is therefore decided in the matrix. The nail's condition depends on how healthy the cell growth is and whether or not there has been any damage to the matrix, such as from knocks, injury (for example, a nail being shut in the door), poor treatment or an infection. However, as long as the matrix has not been permanently damaged, the effect on the nail is usually only temporary.

Lunula

The **lunula** is also known as the half moon. It is found on all nails, but on some it is easier to see. It is at the base of the nails and is the visible part of the matrix.

Nail bed

The **nail bed** is the healthy soft tissue underneath the nail plate. It gives the nail its pink appearance. It contains blood vessels and nerve endings. Ridges in the nail bed help to keep the nail firmly in place as it grows.

Nail plate

The nail plate lies on top of the nail bed and is the main part of the nail. It is pink in colour because of the soft tissue underneath, which is visible through the plate. The nail plate is made up of layers of fat, moisture and growth cells, and these give the nail its strength. If you tear part of the nail off, it is very painful because it is attached to blood vessels and nerve endings.

Free edge

The free edge is the hardest part of the nail. It grows past the end of the nail bed and fingertip. It is whitish in colour, as it has grown beyond the pink tissue. If you break this part of the nail, it does not hurt because it is not joined to blood vessels or nerve endings.

Nail grooves or nail wall

The **nail grooves** are deep ridges that lie along the back and sides of the nail. The grooves at the side of the nail guide the direction of the nail growth. The grooves also help to stop germs from entering the nail bed. If the nail grooves are not kept soft and well-moisturised, hangnails can appear.

These are dry strips of skin at the sides of the nail that can become very sore and **inflamed** if left untreated or pulled off.

Cuticle

The **cuticle** is found at the base of the nail. It is designed to protect the matrix against germs by forming a barrier. You should never cut the cuticle off during a manicure, as the matrix could become infected.

Anatomy and physiology for nail treatments (2)

The nails

Nail health

The state of your nails can provide the secret to your health. A doctor can often tell what illness a person has by looking at the appearance of the nails. For example, some nail conditions can show that a person has heart problems, poor circulation or a lack of iron.

Nail facts

1 The nails are held together with fats and moisture. You can peel back one or two layers when the nails are out of condition.

2 Nails dry out as we get older.

3 The ridges on a nail are natural and are there to help the nail plate stick to the **nail bed**. If the nails are filed or buffed to get a smooth look, this will weaken the nail. However, very deep ridges can be a sign of illness.

4 Fingernails take 3 to 6 months to grow from root to tip.

5 Toenails take 10 to 12 months to grow from root to tip.

6 On average, nails grow one eighth of an inch (0.3 cm) per month.

7 Nails grow faster in the summer than in the winter.

8 If a person is right-handed, his or her fingernails will grow faster on the right hand than on the left hand. This is because the person's right hand gets more stimulation. (The reverse is true for left-handed people.)

9 Men's nails grow faster than women's nails.

10 The longer the finger, the faster the nail growth.

11 Of the nails on the hand, the smallest fingernail grows the slowest, and the thumb nail grows the second slowest.

12 Nails grow faster in younger people.

13 If we restrict our diet too much, our nail growth slows down.

14 If left to grow too long, the nails start to curl.

>> **Get up and go!**

Describe how you think your hands and nails should look when giving a treatment, so that a client will not be put off but will feel confident that she is being treated by a person who knows what she is doing.

Bones of the hand and wrist

There are three sections to the bones of the hand and wrist. These are:

- the carpals in the wrist, consisting of eight bones
- the metacarpals in the hand or palm – there is one metacarpal on each finger and thumb
- the phalanges in the fingers and thumbs – there are three phalanges that make up each finger and two phalanges on the thumb.

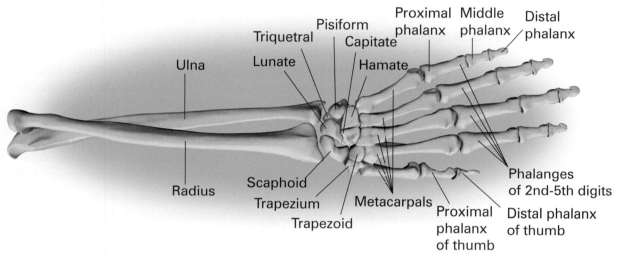

The bones of the hand and wrist

> ### ? Memory jogger
>
> 1 What is the function of the nail plate?
>   A Secretion
>   B Protection
>   C Absorption
>   D Excretion
> 2 Where would you find the lunula?
>   A At the tips of the nails
>   B At the sides of the nails
>   C At the base of the nails
>   D Under the nails
> 3 What is a hangnail?
>   A A split nail
>   B A broken nail
>   C An infected nail
>   D A strip of skin
> 4 What are the three sections to the bones of the hands and wrists?

Treatment times and prices

Cost effectiveness and commercial viability

The commercially acceptable treatment time is the time that you need to take to carry out a treatment, from the client consultation process through to the aftercare advice, while still making money for the salon.

If you take longer than the time that is commercially acceptable to complete a treatment during your assessment, you will not pass because you will not be competent.

If you took too long to complete all your treatments, you wouldn't be able to fit many treatments into one day. You would therefore fail to make much money for the business and this would be commercially unacceptable. When you are working in a salon you should keep to the correct times. If you don't, you will fit in fewer clients – for example, just three instead of six in one day. This will mean the salon will lose money and clients will be kept waiting. Not being commercially viable could mean that your manager decides that you need a course of re-training to bring your skills up to speed and the worst case scenario if you still didn't improve is that you could lose your job. So you can see how important completing the job in the correct time is!

Although it is better for a client not to be rushed out after her treatment, it is not a good idea to leave the client too long in the treatment room once the treatment has finished. This would mean that the treatment room is not available for the next client, and that the therapist is late in starting her next treatment. This delay could then have a knock-on effect for the rest of the day. By the time the last client is seen, the therapist could be an hour or so behind schedule.

To avoid the treatment room being held up in this way, the best solution is to have a relaxing area where a client can sit quietly and have a drink after her treatment. Alternatively, if the salon is large and has many treatment rooms, then it is possible that the next treatment could start in a different room while the client is left to relax where she is.

Recommended treatment times for Level 1 Certificate (NVQ/SVQ) in Beauty therapy

Service (excluding consultation and preparation)	Max time (mins)	Previous time (mins)
Assist with facial skin care treatments	30	45
Assist with nail services	30	30
Apply day make-up	30	New

Salon pricing

Pricing for beauty treatments and services vary from UK regions and town and city areas. Depending on the popularity of the area or type of salon, prices may be up to double the amount of that in another place. So it is difficult to state how much a client would expect to pay for a treatment.

 Get up and go!

1 Choose six towns in the UK.
2 Research the salons offering make-up treatments in the six towns by using a search engine and typing in 'beauty salons in <name of the place>'.
3 When you have your search results click on one of the salons, and see if they have a downloadable brochure which gives the list of treatments they offer and the prices. If not they may just list their prices on their website.
4 Do this until you have six prices for a treatment of your choice.
5 Print off the brochures and highlight the treatments.

 Get ahead

- Create a graph to show the range of prices.
- Compare the prices and show the results to your class group. Discuss your findings.

Index

Index